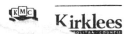

Aromatherapy
for Your Child

Aromatherapy for Your Child

Essential oil remedies for children of all ages

VALERIE ANN WORWOOD

Thorsons

Thorsons
An Imprint of HarperCollins*Publishers*
77-85 Fulham Palace Road
Hammersmith, London W6 8JB

The Thorsons website address is:
www.thorsons.com

First published 2001

10 9 8 7 6 5 4 3 2 1

© Valerie Ann Worwood 2001

Valerie Ann Worwood asserts the moral right to be identified as the author of this work

A catalogue record for this book is available from the British Library

ISBN 0 00 710914 8

Illustrations by Jackie Harland

Printed and bound in Great Britain by Scotprint

Special thanks go to all the parents who have trusted my judgements and advice, brought their children to my practice, used my books for healing, and passed on the information to friends and family, often at school gates and playgrounds. Most of them I have never met, but they have kindly written to me over the years, to tell me their personal stories and to pass on valuable comments.

Contents

Foreword

Nothing in the world is more precious to us than our children, and it's a daunting responsibility to care for them. We all rely heavily on the medical professions, and we should continue to take advantage of all the benefits modern medicine can offer us. But there are times when no help is available, when we have to fall back on our own resources and take the care of our children into our own hands.

Some of us may simply prefer to use natural medicines whenever we can. There is certainly a trend towards natural medicine, not only among the general public but also within the medical professions. The advantages of integrative medicine are increasingly appreciated, as natural remedies are used alongside conventional medical treatment.

There's nothing new in natural medicine. From earliest times parents around the world have taken from nature the herbs and plants they needed to care for the health of their children. Aromatherapy is a modern version of that long tradition of using what is available, and what is natural, and what works. These days we have scientific papers to back up empirical evidence, and instead of long treks into the countryside to collect healing plants we have convenient dropper bottles full of healing essential oils from plants. Aromatherapy offers great convenience and flexibility, and there's never been a better time to take advantage of nature's fragrant pharmacy.

In my practice as a clinical aromatherapist I've seen the wonderful healing effect that aromatherapy and essential oils have on children. Friends and family have used my knowledge, and passed it on to their friends and family, and I constantly hear of the positive results this has brought to both adults and children. Also, readers all over the world who have used the information in my books kindly write and tell me how much aromatherapy has helped them or their children. I'm also a consultant to the aromatherapists working with The Children's Society in England to relieve the difficulties faced by physically or mentally disadvantaged children. They have hills to climb, and aromatherapy helps them.

I did not plan to write a book for children – and I had to think long and hard. There have been suggestions that aromatherapy should only be used by people trained in the profession. Part of this argument maintains that general readers aren't capable of following instructions, and that they shouldn't be encouraged to get involved in something they know nothing about.

As I was about to lift up the receiver and turn down the offer, the phone rang. It was my brother. The previous evening he'd gone to a dinner party where another guest had said that aromatherapy had saved her child's life. Her baby was born prematurely and had severe health difficulties. The doctor at the hospital said there was nothing further they could do, that she should take her baby home and prepare for the worst. The mother was devastated. Then a nurse came and showed her a copy of an aromatherapy book and said, "Go and buy a copy and follow the instructions." She did this, and the baby is now a healthy two-year-old. "What was the book?" someone at the party had asked, and the woman had replied, "*The Fragrant Pharmacy*" – one of my earlier books. When my brother told the woman that I was his sister, she asked him to tell me, "Thanks". *That's* why he had called.

It was like a message saying that aromatherapy can be beneficial to a child's health, and if people know about it they can use it to help their child. So, I offer you here my knowledge, but there's another side to this – you, the carer. You're the person who is going to carry out the instructions, and I rely on you to follow them correctly. Also, please take care to find a reputable supplier of essential oils. If you do both these things, I have confidence that you, too, will discover the healing power of essential oils.

When I was a little girl my mother treated everyday ailments with herbs and healing plants, which were administered around the kitchen table. The tradition of natural medicine lives on in modern aromatherapy. Those of us who have been using essential oils for a long time, and have seen our children grow up, and even have children of their own, take great pleasure in the fact that the younger generations now use essential oils. We recommend them to their friends ... who recommend them to their family and friends, and so on. One drop of essential oil, performing some task of healing, falls into the pool of general knowledge and ripples out, touching others. This is how aromatherapy is today. The ripples are getting stronger, and spreading further, because essential oils work.

But, as a clinical aromatherapist myself, and working with others in the field, I know that individual children can benefit from aromatherapy – children of all ages, temperament and state of health. I finally came to the conclusion that it would be wrong of me not to share the knowledge from which so many others have benefited. Everything in aromatherapy is natural, a gift from God. The essential goodness of essential oils cannot be denied. They are powerful, that is true, and we must always regard them with respect. If we do that, they will help us through some of the hardest times we shall have to face – when our precious children are not well.

What's so Great About Aromatherapy?

Probably every parent has been in the position of having a sick child to care for, but no available help. It's a horrible feeling. Perhaps the doctor is not able to visit until the morning, or you are snowed in and can't go and get help yourself. Using essential oils, however, you can often deal with things when they happen. You're not helpless – there's something you can do; something that's been shown to work through long-term use, and through a great deal of scientific research. And, as well as helping out in emergencies, aromatherapy lets you think proactively about the long-term health of your child.

The essential oils used in aromatherapy are 100 per cent pure, natural essences, distilled from a variety of plants. These are very concentrated substances, which are measured in drops, using just one drop is not unusual. The oils come from flowers, leaves, roots, resin, seeds, fruits and wood, depending on the plant species.

The first essential oil people often buy is lavender, because it's so versatile. It can help with the healing process of cuts and grazes, and is the best thing for burns; plus it smells nice and can be diffused around the home, or put in the bath for when you want to relax and have a good sleep. That's just one oil, but when two or more essential oils are mixed together, they make a new therapeutic composition, which is able to perform tasks not possible with individual oils on their own. Combining essential oils into unique blends gives aromatherapy depth and richness – and tremendous flexibility.

You will discover that the healing power of nature, in the form of aromatherapy, is very easy to use at home. Because the essential oils come in volatile liquid form, there are lots of ways they can be used, and many different heating and diluting methods. The oils come in tiny portable bottles, and don't take up much space. The only extra things you need are a few small empty bottles, some carrier oil, such as almond, and a diffuser. Most other things you might need are likely to be in your home already.

In terms of therapeutic potency, most essential oils have a 'shelf life' of around two years, while after six months the therapeutic properties of the citrus oils, like lemon, are said to be diminished. But even when an essential oil has lost its therapeutic vibrancy, it can still be used in all sorts of ways. Lemon, for example, can be used in a room diffuser or air-freshening spray, and even to wipe down kitchen surfaces, or to freshen up the laundry.

There's no way of telling when a child might get sick. They can walk out of their bed in the middle of the night and complain of sudden earache, or just as easily wake up with a cough. With aromatherapy, it's often possible to deal with the situation right there and then, which is a great relief when you have a crying child asking for your help. Essential oils won't be able to assist with every crisis you'll have to deal with as a parent, but they can probably deal with more than you think they can. As you discover this fact, you will wonder how you ever managed before.

ONE

The Essentials

By reading this chapter from beginning to end, you'll know some of the basics about using home-help aromatherapy for children. The A–Z of conditions (Chapter 8) contains instructions on the use of essential oils for different medical problems. When using essential oils for children more generally, there are general directions and information you need to have.

 Essential oils are pure plant essences. They're distilled from flowers, leaves, seeds, fruit, roots, resin and wood. See Chapter 2.

 Only some essential oils are suitable for children. The chart on pages 4–6 shows which oils you can use, according to the child's age.

 Essential oils, when used correctly, do not conflict with medically prescribed drugs. They can be used alongside other treatments. Integrative medicine is the way of the future.

 Essential oils are used externally, that is, on the outside of the body. Use them in body oils, lotions, creams, gels, baths, showers, foot baths, compresses, dressings, and in the sponging-down method. You can diffuse them in the atmosphere, spray them in the air or inhale them from a tissue (see pages 9–18).

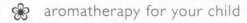

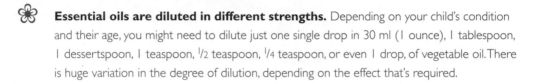 **Essential oils are diluted in different strengths.** Depending on your child's condition and their age, you might need to dilute just one single drop in 30 ml (1 ounce), 1 tablespoon, 1 dessertspoon, 1 teaspoon, $^1\!/_2$ teaspoon, $^1\!/_4$ teaspoon, or even 1 drop, of vegetable oil. There is huge variation in the degree of dilution, depending on the effect that's required.

Blend two or more essential oils together before diluting. When using two or more essential oils, mix them all together in the empty bottle so they can amalgamate well, then add the carrier oil on top. When using a single essential oil, it doesn't matter if you put it in the bottle before or after the carrier oil.

Sometimes we use just 1 or 2 drops of a complex mix of essential oils. Blends of many oils are often more potent than single oils. In those blends, some essential oils might contribute 1 or 2 drops, while others are needed in larger amounts (say, 5 or 6 drops). A mix is made up of both different essential oils and different amounts of essential oil. When the mix is complete, we can take from it how much we need. This may be just 1 drop – but it will be a complex drop that combines many properties.

We often prepare more diluted oil than we intend to use. For example, in the case of baby's colic, only 1 drop of colic mix is needed in $^1\!/_2$ teaspoon of vegetable oil. Of this, only a very small amount will be used; the rest will go to waste. However, there's no other way to do it: you can't measure less than 1 drop of essential oil easily at home, so to get the right essential-oil-to-vegetable oil ratio, we have to make more than we need.

Essential oils, and diluted blends, are delicate. Keep all pure essential oils, and all diluted oils, in a cool, dry, dark place – away from sunlight.

TWO

Essential Oils

Nature's healing tools

Essential oils are distilled from certain healing plants, usually by steam distillation. They are produced all around the world for use in medicine, food, drink, perfumery and, of course, aromatherapy.

Almost all essential oils are antiseptic, and individual oils have their own particular healing characteristics. Some have strong anti-bacterial properties; others are anti-viral, anti-fungal, anti-inflammatory or anti-spasmodic. Some are calming, others are stimulating. Each essential oil has a healing profile (comprised of several characteristics) that is unique to itself.

When using essential oils on children, it's important to recognize that some oils are not suitable for them. That might be because the oil has hormonal properties, or it may be too powerful for the child's weaker constitution. If using essential oil for a particular condition, only use the oils recommended in that section of the A–Z of conditions (Chapter 8). For more general purposes, use the essential oils recommended for your child's age group, as outlined in the chart on pages 4–6.

What's in a name?

The name of essential oils is very important. There are many different types of eucalyptus or chamomile, for example, each with its own particular healing properties. When I recommend chamomile roman, don't confuse it with chamomile german, or with ormenis flower, which some people call chamomile maroc. Please take care to use the correct essential oil for the job; this is especially important in the case of children. Thyme oil is not generally recommended for children because it is so strong, but there's an alternative in the related thyme linalol, which is excellent for use on children. Due to the growth of aromatherapy, there are now many good suppliers of pure essential oil, who can supply you with the essential oil you need, often by mail order.

Child's age	Essential oils	Basic carrier oils	Small additions – base oils
Newborn	chamomile roman, chamomile german, lavender, mandarin, dill	almond (sweet)	jojoba, wheatgerm
2–6 months	chamomile roman, chamomile german, lavender, mandarin, dill, eucalyptus radiata, neroli, tea tree, geranium, rose otto	almond (sweet)	jojoba, wheatgerm
7 months–1 year	chamomile roman, chamomile german, lavender, mandarin, dill, eucalyptus radiata, neroli, tea tree, geranium, rose otto, palmarosa, petitgrain, niaouli, tangerine, cardamom	almond (sweet)	jojoba, wheatgerm, calendula – infusion
2–5 years	chamomile roman, chamomile german, lavender, mandarin, dill, eucalyptus radiata, neroli, tea tree, geranium, rose otto, palmarosa,		

	petitgrain, niaouli, tangerine, cardamom, thyme linalol, ginger, lemon, grapefruit, ravensara, ormenis flower, coriander, helichrysum, yarrow	almond (sweet)	jojoba, wheatgerm, calendula – infusion, red carrot
6–8 years	chamomile roman, chamomile german, lavender, mandarin, dill, eucalyptus radiata, neroli, tea tree, geranium, rose otto, palmarosa, petitgrain, niaouli, tangerine, cardamom, thyme linalol, ginger, lemon, grapefruit, ravensara, ormenis flower, coriander, helichrysum, yarrow, bergamot, marjoram, eucalyptus citriodora, myrtle, pine, ho-wood, myrrh, spikenard, orange	almond (sweet), apricot. peach kernel, camellia, sunflower, grapeseed	jojoba, wheatgerm, calendula – infusion, red carrot
9–11 years	chamomile roman, chamomile german, lavender, mandarin, dill, eucalyptus radiata, neroli, tea tree, geranium, rose otto, palmarosa, petitgrain, niaouli, tangerine, cardamom, thyme linalol, ginger, lemon, grapefruit, ravensara, ormenis flower, coriander, helichrysum, yarrow, bergamot, marjoram, eucalyptus citriodora, myrtle, pine, ho-wood, myrrh, spikenard, orange, frankincense, cypress, melissa, elemi, ylang-ylang	almond (sweet), apricot, peach kernel, camellia, sunflower, grapeseed	jojoba, wheatgerm, calendula – infusion, red carrot

| 12–15 years | chamomile roman, chamomile german, lavender, mandarin, dill, eucalyptus radiata, neroli, tea tree, geranium, rose otto, palmarosa, petitgrain, niaouli, tangerine, cardamom, thyme linalol, ginger, lemon, grapefruit, ravensara, ormenis flower, coriander, helichrysum, yarrow, bergamot, marjoram, eucalyptus citriodora, myrtle, pine, ho-wood, myrrh, spikenard, orange, frankincense, cypress, melissa, elemi, ylang-ylang | almond (sweet), apricot, peach kernel, camellia, sunflower, grapeseed | jojoba, wheatgerm, calendula – infusion, red carrot |

Room method oils

With children, the following essential oils can only be used in the room methods (such as diffusers and sprays). Unless otherwise indicated in this book, only use with children over 3 years of age.

oregano	thyme red	clove	cinnamon
citronella	fennel	bay	

Buying and storing

If you are planning to use essential oils with children, it is crucial to find a good supplier of pure essential oils – organic if possible. Many of the ranges of essential oil sold today are not what they seem. They could be chemical copies of essential oil, made to mimic the aroma, or industrial-quality essential oils, which are too old to have any therapeutic qualities left. They might be pure oils, but diluted in a vegetable oil already – and not suitable for the purposes outlined in this book. Some are sold as 'fragrant oils' or even 'aromatherapy oils', and are intended for use as sweet-smelling body oils, or as room fragrances. But you need the essential oils as healing tools.

Most health stores will sell 100 per cent pure essential oil, and if you have any difficulty look at the small ads in health magazines, where mail-order suppliers are likely to be found.

Essential oils should be supplied in dark glass bottles that have a dropper-stopper. Always read the label carefully, to check that it says '100 per cent pure essential oil'. Ideally, the Latin name should be printed on the label, along with a 'sell-by' date – which might be two years away.

Keep your essential oils and blends somewhere dark, cool and away from a humid atmosphere. Bathrooms are often full of damp steam, so are not a good place to keep them. Specially made wooden storage boxes are available, and are the most convenient way to store the essential oils. You also need to put the oils somewhere where they can't be reached by inquisitive little minds and hands, perhaps on a high shelf.

THREE

Using Essential Oils

The methods

There are two ways to use aromatherapy on children. You can use essential oils to get a child well – which is a home-help form of clinical aromatherapy, and is the main subject of this book; aromatherapy can be also be used simply to give a general sense of well-being (which is never far from our minds) – this is elaborated upon in Chapter 6.

All essential oils should be sold with a dropper-hole insert already in place, which makes measuring easy. Essential oils differ in terms of their density and viscosity: the watery type such as lavender come out of the dropper hole easily, while you have to be patient with the syrupy ones such as sandalwood.

In the A–Z of conditions (Chapter 8), there are recommended methods and sometimes particular instructions for the number of drops to use for children of different age groups. Those amounts are very specific for that particular condition, and are never a 'general rule'. There are guidelines for the amount of essential oil that should be used with a child of a particular age, for all the different methods. These are given below.

Baths	**TD Amount to use**	
	Unless following instructions	
	elsewhere in this book	

Instructions

Run the bath as usual, then add the teaspoon of diluted essential oil and swish the water around. Shut the door to keep the aroma in the bathroom. Use essential oils diluted in a small amount of vegetable oil, milk or milk powder.

In baths, diluted essential oils are gentler on children's delicate skin.

	All diluted in 1 teaspoon of vegetable oil	
Up to 6 months	1 drop, then use $1/4$ this amount	
6 months–2 years	1 drop, then use $1/2$ this amount	
2–5 years	1–2 drops, then use $1/2$ this amount	
6–10 years	1–3 drops	
11 years and over	1–4 drops	

Body oil or body rub	**TD Amount to use**	
	Unless following instructions	
	elsewhere in this book	

Instructions

Use the body oil or body rub like a body lotion – just smooth it on the skin. For suggested well-being blends, see Chapter 6.

If using one single essential oil, just add it to the base (vegetable) oil already in the bottle. If using two or more essential oils, put them into the empty bottle first, mix them well by rolling the bottle between your hands, and then pour in the vegetable oil – up to the 'shoulder' (not as far as the neck of the bottle) – then roll again.

See also Chapter 4.

	All diluted in 30 ml (1 ounce) vegetable oil	
Newborns	0–1 drop	
2–6 months	1–2 drops	
6–12 months	1–3 drops	
1–4 years	1–5 drops	
5–7 years	3–6 drops	
8–12 years	5–9 drops	
Puberty	5–10 drops	

Clothing	TD Amount to use
	Unless following instructions
	elsewhere in this book

Instructions

Some essential oils will leave a mark on material, so only use this method if the clothes aren't valuable. It's a useful way of keeping insects at bay. Put neat essential oil or diluted spray on the outside of socks, shoes, the bottoms of shorts, skirts or trouser legs, or on the collar, sleeves or cuffs of shirts and tops.	On children over 5 years only
	1 drop
This method is also useful for students who want to inhale a concentration-enhancing aroma when they're taking an exam – put it on the cuff of a long-sleeved shirt.	

Compresses	TD Amount to use
	Unless following instructions
	elsewhere in this book

Instructions

Put 1/2 pint water in a bowl, and add the essential oil (alternatively, use hydrolats or essential oil 'waters' – see page 18).	On children over 2 years only
	2–4 drops
Put the compress material in the water and leave it to soak until throroughly soaked with the compress mixture. Then squeeze out the excess water, and place the compress over the area.	
Hold or tie it in place.	

Eye compresses should only be made with hydrolats or 'waters', taking care that no substance gets into the eye.

Always use 100 per cent natural material, unbleached if possible, and large enough to cover the affected area when folded several times.

Compresses can be used hot, warm, tepid, cool or cold. Warmth increases the flow of blood to an area, whereas cold restricts the flow of blood to an area.

Cotton bud

TD   Amount to use
Unless following instructions
elsewhere in this book

Instructions

Put the undiluted essential oil on to a wet cotton bud, and apply directly to the affected area.

On children over 2 years only

Diffusers/burners

TD   Amount to use
Unless following instructions
elsewhere in this book

Instructions

Diffusers/burners are two-tier objects, with a top bowl-like section for the water and essential oil, and a lower section for the tea-light candle, which heats the water above. Put warm water in the upper bowl, light the candle below, then place your chosen essential oil(s) on to the water.

Up to 2 years	1–2 drops
2–5 years	1–3 drops
6–10 years	1–4 drops
11 and over	1–5 drops

As the candle heats the water, the essential oils and water evaporate. Keep an eye on diffusers to make sure the water does not evaporate before the candle goes out. If the water level is looking low, top it up with more warm water.

Diffusers are usually made of ceramic or glass. If ceramic, make sure the water-bowl area is glazed – so you can wipe it with a cloth between use and clear away any gooey residue.

There are also electrical diffusers/burners, with no candle section. Make sure you do not leave these plugged in after the water has evaporated.

Nebulizers or oil vaporizers put a continuous fine spray of essential oil into the atmosphere. They were designed for clinical use and should not be used at home for children, as the amount of essential oil emitted (and inhaled) is far too high.

Dressings

TD   Amount to use
Unless following instructions
elsewhere in this book

Instructions

This method is used to help stop the spread of infection and to promote the healing of wounds. The essential oil is put directly on to the dressing covering the affected area – such as plasters (the inner, fabric part) or lint and gauze dressing. Leave the essential oil to dry before applying; this will prevent it stinging, but will still be effective.

On children over 2 years only
1–2 drops

Face oils	**TD**	**Amount to use**
		Unless following instructions
		elsewhere in this book

Instructions

Face oils should only be used if there is a condition	All diluted in 15 ml (¹/₂ ounce) almond oil	
that requires it.	Up to 2 years	1 drop
	3–5 years	1–3 drops
Avoid the eye, mouth and nose areas.	6-10 years	1–4 drops
	11 and over	1–6 drops

Foot baths	**TD**	**Amount to use**
		Unless following instructions
		elsewhere in this book

Instructions

Fill a large bowl with warm water and add 1 teaspoon of	All diluted in 1 teaspoon vegetable oil	
diluted essential oil, swishing it around before placing the	On children over 2 years only	
feet in the bowl.	2–5 years	1 drop
	6–10 years	1–2 drops
	11 and over	1–3 drops

Humidifiers	TD Amount to use Unless following instructions elsewhere in this book
Instructions Add the essential oil to the water in the humidifier. Essential oils can leave a sticky residue. This should not be a problem with the type of humidifier that hangs over radiators; however, the more complex electrical types should be assessed before use, to see whether any sticky essential oil residue migh	Any age 1–4 drops per pint of water

Inhalation	TD Amount to use Unless following instructions elsewhere in this book
Instructions *Tissue or handkerchief method* Put the essential oil on to a paper tissue or cotton handkerchief, and sniff from it when required.	On children over 2 years only 1–2 drops
Pillow method This method is usually used to assist breathing or sleeping. Put the essential oil on a corner of the pillow – on the underside, and away from the eyes. Some essential oils stain material – so use an old pillowcase. Alternatively, put the essential oil on a cotton-wool ball and put it inside the pillowcase – somewhere where it will be away from the eyes.	On children over 6 months only 1–2 drops

Pyjama method

Before your child is ready for bed, put a drop of essential oil on the pyjamas, and allow it to dry.

Put it at the back – on the collar, the back area or on the chest.

On children over 6 months only

1 drop

Lotions, creams and gels

TD Amount to use
Unless following instructions
elsewhere in this book

Instructions

Essential oils can be diluted in materials other than vegetable oils. Use an unperfumed lotion, cream or gel that is made of natural materials.

Add the required number of essential oil drops suitable for the age of the child, then mix well.

All diluted in 30 ml (1 ounce) lotion/cream/gel.

Up to 6 months	0–1 drop
6–12 months	1–2 drops
1–4 years	1–5 drops
5–7 years	3–6 drops
8–12 years	5–9 drops

Room sprays

TD Amount to use
Unless following instructions
elsewhere in this book

Instructions

Put the warm water in a new plant-mister, and add the essential oil. Shake it vigorously, then spray high into the air. Avoid spraying over anything that could be damaged if the water droplets fall on it – such as wooden furniture or delicate materials.

On children over 3 months only

10 drops to each 1/2 pint lukewarm water

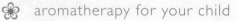

Showers

TD Amount to use
Unless following instructions
elsewhere in this book

Instructions

Only use the essential oils of chamomile, lavender or geranium with this method.

On children over 5 years only
1–2 drops

Put the essential oil on a dry washcloth, wet it thoroughly with water, then wipe the washcloth over the body while the shower is running.

Avoid the face and genital areas.

Sponging down

TD Amount to use
Unless following instructions
elsewhere in this book

Instructions

Put 2 pints warm or lukewarm water in a bowl. Add the essential oil, and swish around well. Use the water to sponge down your child.

On children over 1 year only
1–5 years   3 drops
6–10 years   4 drops

Wash

TD   Amount to use
Unless following instructions
elsewhere in this book

Instructions

Put the water in a bottle, add the essential oils, and shake well. Then pour though a paper coffee-filter and rebottle.

On children over 1 year only

20 drops in 1 pint warm water

This prepared wash is useful for washing infected or other areas, such as cuts and grazes.

Water bowl

TD   Amount to use
Unless following instructions
elsewhere in this book

Instructions

Put 1 pint boiling water into a heatproof bowl, and take it to the room where it is needed. Add the essential oil to the steaming water.

Place the bowl in an area of the room where children and animals cannot reach

All diluted in 1 pint water

Up to 2 years	1–2 drops
2–5 years	1–3 drops
6–10 years	1–4 drops
11 and over	1–5 drops

Hydrolats, essential oil 'waters' and infused oils

Throughout this book I refer to hydrolats, essential oil 'waters' and infused oils. These are all products which include some elements of the healing properties of the essential oils found in plants. Hydrolats can't be made at home, but can be purchased from specialist suppliers; essential oil 'waters' are made with essential oils and water, and can be used in place of hydrolats; and infused oils can be purchased or made at home.

Hydrolats

A great deal of water is used in the process of essential oil distillation, and is often sold on as a by-product of the manufacturing process as a 'hydrolat'. Rosewater and orange-flower water, which are used in beauty preparations and cooking, are diluted hydrolats. Herbal medicine uses these and other hydrolats, such as lavender, tea tree and chamomile.

Only the water-soluble components in plants become imbued in the water used in the distillation process. Consequently, hydrolats can't be thought of as 'watered-down essential oils' because they don't contain all of the essential oils' components. Hydrolats very often smell quite different to both the plant and the essential oil – lavender and rosemary are good examples.

Hydrolats have antiseptic properties. As well as in compresses, for example, they can be used to spray rooms or bedclothes. They often have a delicious fragrance. Hydrolats have to be bought like an essential oil, and if your supplier doesn't sell them, a herbalist might.

Essential oil 'waters'

The water-infusion method creates an essential oil 'water', and can be used in place of a hydrolat. In a heatproof bowl, pour $^{1}/_{2}$ pint boiling water. Then add 6–10 drops of your chosen essential oil. Cover the bowl completely, so the cooled, condensed water falls back into the water. Then pour the mixture through an unbleached, paper coffee-filter, to take out the globules of essential oil. Leave it to cool, then bottle.

Infused oils

There are two ways to make an infused oil. In the first, you get a jam-jar or other container that can be kept tightly shut, and fill it with whatever plant material you want to use such as lavender, chamomile, marigold or calendula. Use the part of the plant that contains the essential oils – mostly it's in the flowers, although with rosemary you use the spiky leaves. Pack in as much as you can, then fill the jar with a good, organic vegetable oil, such as sunflower, grapeseed or almond. Put the lid on tightly, and put the jar somewhere in the sun, like on the windowsill. Shake the bottle every day. After at least 48 hours, strain the oil again. To really get all the bits out, strain the oil through an unbleached paper coffee-filter. It's thick, so this will take some time. To make the oil stronger, use the same oil and add more fresh plant material, and repeat the process. Carry on until you get the aroma as strong as you want it.

The second method involves putting the flower-heads or other plant material in a jar with the oil (as above) and, after sealing the jar, gently heating the oil and the plant together. This is done by putting the jar into several centimetres of water in a pot, on the cooker. Use a low heat – there should be no bubbling or boiling. Strain as usual.

Other ingredients

The following ingredients have been used throughout this book.

Alcohol

Use only pure, organic, good-quality alcohol, or vodka.

Aloe vera

The aloe vera plant has renowned healing properties. It has long, hard, thick, spiky leaves, in the centre of which is a sticky gel-like substance, which can be taken out and used. The plant grows easily on sunny window ledges, requires little maintenance and propagates itself – producing more baby plants, which can be repotted. The plant provides an easily accessible, fresh source of aloe vera, which is the best form to use. However, aloe vera can also easily be purchased in water or gel form. Aloe vera is an anti-inflammatory, and can soothe the skin and help to heal cuts, grazes and burns, as well as ease insect bites.

Baking soda

Sodium bicarbonate ($NaHCO_3$) – a sodium salt which softens water. When used in the bath, it relieves itching and is soothing to the skin.

Beeswax

Always use the pure, unbleached variety. This is obtainable from health shops, specialist stores, bee-keepers, and from some good-quality drugstores and pharmacies.

Bicarbonate of soda

Sodium carbonate, also known as 'washing soda' (Na_2CO_3).

Calamine lotion

A pink or white pharmaceutical preparation for soothing and calming the skin. It can be found in chemists.

Cider vinegar

This must be organic if used to soothe and soften the skin. It can help restore the acid mantle of the skin and helps soothe irritation and stings.

Colloidal silver

This is a specialized product, with strong anti-bacterial and anti-fungal properties. It is available from good health food shops.

Epsom salts

This is used to help soothe sore muscles and stiffness. It is not a water softener.

Glucose powder

A powdered form of glucose, which is found in most food stores and chemists.

Green clay

This has long been used in European health and beauty preparations. The clay, which is taken directly from the ground, has healing properties. It is deodorizing, and can help skin problems.

Honey

Only use the very best you can find – a pure organic flower honey. Manuka honey is very healing, and is highly recommended for the purposes outlined in this book.

Iodine

Easily found in chemists.

Menthol crystals

This is crystallized menthol, extracted from the mint plant family. It is available from chemists.

Myrrh tincture

Myrrh tincture is an alcoholic solution of myrrh. It's found in chemists.

Oats/oatmeal

Only use raw, organic oats or oatmeal, found in organic food shops, and some supermarkets.

Rose water

Produced in the distillation of rose oil. The most concentrated form is a 'hydrolat' or, when that is re-diluted, it is called rose water. It's used in cooking and skin care – for its skin-softening and healing properties.

Salt

Salt is healing and cleansing. The salt referred to in this book is either sea salt or rock salt. It should contain as few chemical or additional substances as possible.

Vegetable-based ointment ('Vaseline type')

This is usually available from health/organic food shops, but may be found in some chemists.

Water

When water is mentioned as an ingredient – other than for baths and compresses – it means spring or distilled water.

Witch hazel

Witch hazel is made from a bush, and comes in distilled or infused form. It's a mild astringent with soothing and sting-relieving properties.

Zinc oxide cream

A cream containing zinc that is widely used as a skin-healing medium. Easily available from chemists.

Equipment used

Bottles

Always keep essential oils and blends in dark bottles – brown, green or blue.

Hot-water bottle

This refers to a large, flat rubber bottle which you fill with warm water. It is best to use one with a cover made of fluffy material.

Muslin

Muslin is a very fine cheesecloth-like material. Try to find unbleached muslin – available from specialist material shops and some craft shops.

Paper coffee-filters

This refers to the triangular-shaped papers used to filter coffee. Use the unbleached paper variety.

Warm bags

These contain wheat, corn, buckwheat, rice, cherry stones and other natural materials. They are covered in a material that can be heated in the microwave or put in the refrigerator or freezer, and can be found in many department stores and health food shops.

The Cave Man Eating Plan

Thousands of years ago, when people were first on this planet, there were no sugar-enhanced foods, no quickly prepared foods, no dairy foods or wheat products. We don't know if children were healthier then, but we do know that adopting an eating plan based on the food that humans first ate is good for our children – especially those who have become unhealthy, and subject to pollution-related disorders and oversensitivity to foods.

The Cave Man Eating Plan is very simple. If the food walks, swims or flies, you can eat it. If it grows in the ground or on a tree, you can eat it. If the food is organically grown, you can eat it, and if it's frozen, you can eat it. What you can't eat are pre-cooked or pre-prepared foods, anything in a tin or packet, no sweets, fizzy drinks or artificially flavoured foods.

Cutting these things from the diet is not as hard as it first seems. Meat and fish can be bought fresh or frozen, and cooked with natural herbs or spices. Salt and pepper are allowed. Vegetables can be steamed, roasted, boiled or eaten raw in salads of all types. Desserts can be made from frozen fruit juice – just put it in your blender and whisk it up with honey. Fruit can be eaten raw or baked in pies. Cook those biscuits, but don't use prepared mixes (which may contain chemicals, and will certainly contain preservatives).

If dairy products are needed, get organic milk – which contains nothing but milk. Eat organic butter, which is far better for you than chemically prepared spreads. Use cold-pressed organic oils for cooking. Make your own lollies with pure fruit juice, and your own fizzy drinks with fruit juice and carbonated water.

Organic food may cost you more, but you'll be saving by not buying all that junk food. Get the kids baking. Give them a basic recipe and let their imaginations run wild.

Some children experience withdrawal symptoms after starting the Cave Man Eating Plan, as the chemical flavourings and preservatives are taken away. It's the same as someone giving up cigarettes, alcohol or caffeine – the first few days can be really rough. Your child may be grumpy and irritable, particularly if his or her favourite drink is not allowed. But do persevere with the Cave Man Eating Plan for at least six weeks, and then see if his or her breathing, skin, emotions and behaviour have improved. Does your child seem happier and less aggressive? Does he or she settle into homework more easily? Are there now more cuddles than arguments? After six weeks, you can give your child the occasional treat – a canned drink perhaps, a chocolate bar, some ice cream or a bit of fast food.

Ideally, the whole family should be involved, and should follow the Cave Man Eating Plan, too – to show solidarity and to support the child it's intended for, and also because they will benefit just as much. The rest is up to you. Until our children can make correctly informed food choices at a later age, it is our responsibility to make sure that – seeing as 'You are what you eat' – we feed our children well.

FOUR

Blending

Blending is all about combining essential oils with a carrier oil (sometimes called a base oil or vegetable oil). Essential and carrier oils are blended together in order to dilute the essential oil, allowing it to be spread over a greater area of skin at the low dosages required.

The following list of carrier oils contains only those used in this book. Some are used very often, while others are used only for particular conditions. Carrier oils have their own healing properties and any particular one might be more appropriate for certain conditions than others. Almond oil is by far the most useful carrier oil to have for use on children, as it can be used in nearly all blending situations. Always try to buy the best-quality carrier oils you can find – organic and 'cold-pressed'.

Carrier oils for children

almond
camellia
grapeseed
rosehip seed
sunflower
avocado
castor
jojoba
calendula oil (infused)
evening primrose
olive
St John's Wort (infused)
sesame seed

How much should I use?

To start with, the amount of essential oil and carrier oil you use partly depends on whether you're blending for a baby, infant, child or adolescent. It also makes a difference whether you're blending for the 'caring touch massage', when your child is well; or for a specific ailment when they are not so well. And each condition will require the essential oil to be diluted in different volumes of carrier oil, and at different strengths. So you could say there are no hard-and-fast rules, but there are general guidelines for home use. These are as follows:

Age of child	Number of drops essential oil	Diluted in
Newborn	1–2	30 ml (1 ounce) vegetable oil
2–6 months	1–3	
6–12 months	1–4	
1–4 years	5–8	
5–7 years	5–10	
8–12 years	5–12	
Puberty	10–20	

Two figures feature under 'Number of drops essential oil' above – the minimum and the maximum dosage. For chronic, longstanding conditions, always start with the minimum number of drops and if that doesn't seem to be helping, add an extra drop into the diluted oil until you find the right dosage for your child. The higher numbers are the upper limits recommended, and for acute situations only.

There are no general diluting guidelines for when a child is ill, because there is no such thing as a general illness! Each infection or disorder needs to be treated with essential oils specific to it, by an appropriate method, using a specific amount of essential oil and carrier oil. Across the many different types of medical condition, there's huge variation as to how much essential oil would be used in each situation. Also, how much you use depends on whether the condition has been going on for a long time and is 'chronic', or has only just happened and is 'acute'.

Chronic cases would use lower amounts of essential oil, working upwards (if required) depending on the severity of the condition. There are other factors to consider when deciding how much to use, as well, such as your child's body weight.

Body weight

Throughout this book, suggested amounts of essential oil have been given for the average weight of a child at a certain age. However, as we all know, very few people are average – 'average' is where we meet, not where we are!

The more body fat a child has, the less essential oil can be absorbed into the body where it is needed. So, if your child is over five years of age and he or she is carrying a lot of extra body fat, or is very tall for his or her age, or has a heavy frame, move to the amount recommendations for the next age group.

Organ maturity

One reason different amounts of essential oil are recommended for the different age groups is that children's organs are at different stages of development. Compare the skin of a newborn baby with that of a 10-year-old child, and you'll notice a big difference. The digestive system of a newborn is only mature enough to take the nutrients out of its mother's milk or specially formulated baby milk. As the child gets older, they can eat mashed-up food, but no big pieces, that comes later. And so it is – everything in its own time. You have to be more flexible when using essential oils on children than you do on adults, simply because children are growing and developing.

Acute or chronic?

Acute conditions are those which materialize suddenly and may need first aid, whereas a chronic condition has persisted for a long time. Throughout this book if you see a drops recommendation for a particular condition with two numbers, say, '3–5 drops', use the lower number (3 drops) on people with a chronic condition and, if that isn't effective, add one more drop, see how that works, and so on up to the maximum of 5. If the condition is acute, the higher amount could be used straight away, if appropriate.

Illness/disease condition

Depending on the severity of a condition at any particular time, use the number of drops that seems appropriate choosing between the minimum and maximum drops given.

Storing blends

Put labels on all blends, saying who they were prepared for, for which medical condition, the ingredients – and the date. When you come back some time later, wondering if the oil is still good to use, at least if you put the date on the bottle label, you'll know when it was prepared.

Diluted blends of essential oil should not be kept for a long time – the vegetable carrier oil will go rancid after a while. It's best to only make up the amount of diluted oil you will need to use for the next week or two. Make up fresh oils as you need them.

Carrier oils for children

The following carrier oils have been suggested in different chapters. In general, almond oil is the best to use on babies and children of all ages, so when in doubt use that. Some of the oils listed below might only be mentioned once or twice in the book, because they are not 'everyday' oils but are good to use for specific conditions. Castor oil, for example, is helpful in cases of flaky skin, but you wouldn't use it for very much else.

Essential oils can be diluted in other mediums or 'carriers' as well as in vegetable oils. For a list of these, see Chapter 3.

Almond (sweet nut) oil

This has an emollient, softening and nourishing effects on the skin, and is highly suitable for babies and children.

Avocado (flesh) oil

Use in combination with other carrier oils – use one-third of avocado combined with two-thirds of almond oil, unless otherwise directed in an instruction. Avocado can be found in refined form, or in its unrefined state – thick, and deep green. It's very nourishing to the skin, and contains minerals and vitamins, and is used mainly for dry or flaky skin conditions.

Camellia seed oil

This is used for its skin-softening and -nourishing effects, and for skin problems. It can be used on its own or in combination with other carrier oils.

Castor oil

This is not often used in aromatherapy, but it is useful in small amounts, for flaky skin and scalp conditions.

Evening primrose oil

This is only used as an addition to other carrier oils – and only in very small quantities. It helps to repair damaged skin and keeps the skin healthy.

Grapeseed

This is used on its own, when a more astringent oil is required. It can be difficult to find organic grapeseed oil.

Jojoba oil

This oil is considered to be more of a 'liquid wax', and is very useful for certain conditions. It has a softening effect on the skin and is good for the scalp and hair. Only use small amounts, and in combination with other carrier oils.

Olive oil

This is a good oil to use on dry skin, and on skins that need nourishing. It's a traditional healing oil, but the smell can overpower the aroma of the essential oils. Only use organically grown, cold-pressed, virgin olive oil.

Rosehip seed oil

Use only very small amounts, in combination with other carrier oils. This is a very regenerative healing oil, useful for scarring and for certain skin conditions.

Sesame oil

Sesame plays a big part in traditional healing systems, such as in Indian Ayurvedic healing. It has a very strong odour, which may overpower the essential oils.

Sunflower seed oil

The kind of sunflower oil sold as regular cooking oil is not suitable for the purposes of children's aromatherapy. But organic, cold-pressed sunflower is easily available, and can be used as a carrier oil for children. It has some emollient properties for the skin, and contains essential fatty acids, which can have a beneficial effect.

Infused oils used in this book

Calendula oil

Calendula oil is made from marigold flowers, and has been used for centuries to heal the skin. It's an orange oil – the stronger the colour, the better the oil – and is used for skin and scalp infections. It also helps to reduce scarring.

St John's Wort

This is a red oil, produced in the same way as calendula oil. Although the flowers used are yellow, they turn the oil red – again, the stronger the colour, the better the oil. It is useful for bruises, sprains and swelling.

FIVE

Safety First

These are the essential safety points to remember. Read through the whole list – you need to know all these things in order to use essential oils safely.

Choosing oils

 There's no need to use essential oils on children unless a health condition requires it. Although your child will certainly benefit from massage carried out for general well-being, don't use essential oils as a 'preventative', in the medical sense – apart from in anti-viral or anti-bacterial room sprays and diffusions.

 Only use essential oils recommended for children.

 The essential oils recommended in this book should be used for the purposes indicated. The range of essential oils given here will cover almost everything that you'll need to do.

Going in the sun

 Certain essential oils should not be used before going in the sun, as they may make the skin more sensitive to the sun's ultraviolet rays. They are:

bergamot (*Citrus aurantium, ssp bergamia*)
grapefruit (*Citrus paradisi*)
lemon (*Citrus limon*)
lime (*Citrus limette*)
mandarin (*Citrus reticulata*)
orange (*Citrus aurantium*)
tangerine (*Citrus reticulata*).

Bottles

 Make sure the dropper stops are firmly in place.

 Ensure the tops are screwed on tightly.

 Write the purchase date on new bottles of essential oil, so later you will know more easily how fresh they are.

Storage

 Store your essential oils and blends well out of reach of children.

 Keep essential oils and blends somewhere dark, with a dry atmosphere, and away from any sources of heat, such as radiators.

 The citrus essential oils deteriorate more quickly than other types of essential oil, but you can make them last longer by keeping them in the refrigerator.

Blends

 Before making blends, make sure all the equipment you will use is sterile. You can do this by boiling the equipment or by using baby sterilizing solution.

 Always use thoroughly dry bottles for blends. If you leave even a tiny amount of water in a bottle after washing, or there is a lot of condensation in the air, the blend will deteriorate and go cloudy.

 After making a blend, put a label on the bottle. It should have – the name of the person the blend was prepared for, the complete list of ingredients, and the date it was prepared.

The skin

 Don't use essential oils neat on the skin – unless indicated to do so in the instructions for a particular condition.

 If your child has very sensitive skin, it's wise to do a patch skin test before using any new single oil or blend.

 If you accidentally splash neat essential oil on to your child, simply wash the area well with soap and warm water.

The eyes

 Keep essential oils away from the eyes, whether neat or diluted in any of the methods (such as forehead compresses).

 If an essential oil gets into the eye, neat or diluted, wash the eye very thoroughly with water, or eye solution. Seek medical help if the eye still stings after being washed out.

The mouth

 Essential oils are not to be taken orally (by mouth) by children.

 If you find that your child has accidentally swallowed essential oil in any form, give him or her a large glass of milk to drink, and visit the casualty department of your hospital immediately.

Fire

 Essential oils are flammable, and should be kept away from naked flames.

Solvents

 Some essential oils act as solvents – such as the citrus oils. They can damage wood and delicate fabrics, and take the print off paper.

Epilepsy

 Talk to your child's doctor if you have any concerns about using aromatherapy.

 Don't use the following stimulating oils on children with epilepsy:

camphor (*Cinnamomum camphora*)
hyssop (*Hyssopus officinalis*)
rosemary (*Rosmarinus officinalis*)
sage (*Salvia officinalis*)
sweet fennel (*Foeniculum vulgare*).

However, this list of calming oils is suitable for epileptic children:

chamomile roman (*Anthemis nobilis*)
geranium (*Pelargonium graveolens*)
jasmine (*Jasminum officinale*)
lavender (*Lavandula angustifolia*)
neroli (*Citrus aurantium*)
petitgrain (*Citrus aurantium*)
rose otto (*Rosa damascena*).

If taking medication . . .

If your child is on medication, use only half the amount of essential oil recommended for his or her age group.

SIX

Caring Touch Massage

There's nothing better for any child than the loving and caring touch of a parent. It may be no more than a gentle touch or squeeze of the hand, but it tells the child that he or she is special. A simple stroke on the cheek lets children know they are loved and cared for. When they fall over, we reach out and rub the knee better, or cuddle them in our arms – these are the everyday forms of touch we instinctually use with our children. And they thrive on it.

Research has shown that massage can help children's growth, both physically and emotionally, while experience in premature baby wards in hospitals shows that touch, even the touch of a single finger, can make a difference to the health of a child. The evidence is mounting – children need a caring touch.

There can be no better way to promote health in your children than to give them regular massages, and you don't need to take a two-year degree course to learn how to do it. You're not going to need any deep-tissue massage techniques, just use very gentle stroking movements. Even with a light touch massage, your hands will move around your child's body, and the first rule of massage is always to work towards the heart, because that's the way the blood flows. All this means in practical terms is that your hands need to work from wrist to shoulder, and ankle to thigh. Good areas to massage are the back, upper abdomen, legs, feet, arms and hands.

Essential oils are a bonus when it comes to massage. They provide great fragrances, they're natural and healthy, and can uplift the spirit. To make a massage oil, all you need is a clean, empty 1-ounce bottle, the carrier oil and your essential oils. Use the following amount of essential oil (according to your child's age) in 30 ml (1 ounce) vegetable carrier oil – almond is best.

Diluted in 30 ml (1 ounce) vegetable oil, e.g. almond

Child's age	Number of drops essential oil
Newborn	1–2
2–6 months	1–3
6–12 months	1–4
1–4 years	5–8
5–7 years	5–10
8–12 years	5–12

Only use a small amount of diluted oil per massage.
Use less, rather than more.

You could use a single oil of your choice or use a blend. When using a single oil, all you have to do is put the essential oil drop or drops into the bottle of almond oil. When making blends, you mix the essential oils together first, to get the blend right. From this, you take the appropriate number of essential oil drops you need, depending upon the age of your child, and put them in the almond or other carrier oil. I find the best way to blend the essential oil and carrier together is to roll the bottle between the palms of your hands.

Here are a few blends that will give pleasure to both you and your child.

The caring touch massage has an additional bonus – aromatic bonding. Whatever aroma you use to massage your child will be associated in his or her mind with relaxing, special times with you. And, the more regular your massages, the stronger that association will be. If the child smells the same aroma in another context (away from the place of massage), he or she will be reminded of the massage and the emotions that went with it – comfort, reassurance and relaxation. This is a smell-bond between you and your child; something that reminds the child of you, and vice versa.

This aromatic bonding can be used to comfort a small child, especially one newly separated from his or her parents – on the first day of starting nursery school, for example. Small children often have to be unwillingly separated from their parents and can feel insecure and even afraid. So, to ease the discomfort of separation, this aromatic link between you and your child can be used. Smear a little of the essential oil you use in your caring touch massage oil, and dab it on a tissue or cotton handkerchief, so your child can smell it during the day. If your child is very young, the carer could just hold the tissue briefly under his or her nose. The aroma should remind your child of you, and give some comfort and reassurance. The message of the massage lives on.

Caring touch massage blends

Mix the essential oils together, then use the correct number of drops for your child's age group, diluted in almond oil.

Sleepy-time
lavender – 4 drops
chamomile roman – 2 drops

Refreshing
lemon – 3 drops
petitgrain – 2 drops

Angelic
rose otto – 3 drops
neroli – 2 drops

Flowery
mandarin – 4 drops
geranium – 2 drops

Calming
petitgrain – 2 drops
neroli – 3 drops

SEVEN

The Basic Care Kit for Children

This kit contains information about the 12 most useful essential oils to have in the home – with these oils, most conditions can be dealt with effectively. There are other oils of course, which are very useful, particularly for certain conditions. These are what you might call the 'extras' – the ones I would want in the home, if I already had the 12 core oils. A basic care kit also needs some carrier oil, and a few small, clean, empty bottles. Most of the equipment you may need is probably in your home already, such as cotton wool, plasters, dressings and a bowl. The only extra thing you may need is a diffuser. Now you're all set.

With the basic tools of aromatherapy, you can take your children's basic care kit even further and make things for the first-aid cupboard. At the end of this chapter you'll find recipes for making your own anti-infectious air spray, first-aid washing mix, antiseptic skin spray, antiseptic anti-fungal powder, herbal healing infused oils, natural ointments and salves, antiseptic ointment, chest congestion ointment, baby oil and baby powder.

First, though, let us look at our children's basic care kit, the 12 most useful essential oils to have in the home for children, with the ailments the oils can help towards healing – either singly or when in combination with others. It may be that the essential oil helps, not with the condition itself, but with one or more of the symptoms; in which case, refer to the section concerned in Chapter 8, the A–Z of conditions.

These essential oils are not listed in any particular order. Which oils you'll find most useful will depend on the age of your child, and the condition they have now or the ailments they are prone to.

Basic care kit – essential oils

Lavender (*Lavandula angustifolia*)

(anti-infectious; anti-bacterial; anti-inflammatory)

cuts, grazes, burns, promotes wound healing, psoriasis, eczema, sunburn, insect bites, headache, migraine, insomnia, rashes, nervous conditions, anxiety, tension

Tea tree (*Melaleuca alternifolia*)

(anti-infectious; anti-bacterial; anti-microbial; anti-fungal; anti-inflammatory)

rashes, insect bites, nail fungus, ringworm, thrush, head lice, sore throats, boils, bronchial congestion, scabies, ulcers, wounds, cold sores, thrush, acne, bronchitis

Chamomile roman (*Anthemis nobilis*)

(anti-bacterial; anti-inflammatory; anti-spasmodic)

pain relief, fevers, skin problems rashes, eczema, teething pain, muscular spasm, calming, helps nervousness, pain relief, insomnia, constipation

Chamomile german (*Matricaria recutita*)

(anti-inflammatory; anti-spasmodic; antibacterial)

skin problems, asthma, eczema, arthritis, acne, ulcerations, fever, wound healing, nervousness, digestive complaints

Thyme linalol (*Thymus vulgaris, type linalol*)

(anti-bacterial; anti-viral; anti-infectious; anti-fungal)

all infections; including viral, mucus congestion, colds, flu, muscular pain, arthritis, bronchitis, pneumonia, tuberculosis, thrush, coughs, throat infections, warts, pain relief

Ravensara (*Ravensara aromatica*)

(anti-viral; anti-bacterial; anti-infectious)

colds, flu, bronchitis, diarrhoea, fever, cold sores, sinusitis, whooping cough, herpes, chickenpox, measles, muscular pain, swollen lymph glands

Niaouli (*Melaleuca quinquenervia/viridiflora*)

(anti-bacterial, anti-parasitic, anti-infectious, anti-viral)

colds, coughs, bronchitis, sinusitis

Cardamom (*Elettaria cardamomum*)

(anti-spasmodic)

indigestion, flatulence, muscular cramps, fatigue, muscular spasms, catarrh, sinus headaches, constipation

Mandarin (*Citrus reticulata*)

(anti-spasmodic)

convalescence, digestive problems, nervous tension, irritability, constipation, insomnia, anxiety

Eucalyptus radiata (*Eucalyptus radiata*)

(anti-infectious, anti-bacterial, anti-inflammatory)

bronchitis, catarrh, coughs, colds, flu, fever, sinusitis, headaches, asthma, insect bites, rashes, acne

Helichrysum (*Helichrysum angustifolium;* also called everlasting or immortelle)

(analgesic; anti-bacterial)

bronchitis, analgesic, pain relief, bruising, coughs, arthritis, circulation problems

Petitgrain (*Citrus aurantium*)

(anti-spasmodic)

spots, boils, nervousness, insomnia, anxiety, stress, calming

'Extra' basic care kit essential oils

Aside from the 12 listed above, there are other essential oils that are also very useful to have in your children's basic care kit. I've listed them in order of preference – by which I mean that, if I had to choose the most useful, the one at the top of the list would come first; and the second oil listed would be the next most useful, and so on:

geranium (*Pelargonium graveolens*)
palmarosa (*Cymbopogon martinii*)
manuka (*Leptospermum scoparium*)
neroli (*Citrus aurantium*)
rosemary (*Rosmarinus officinalis*)
lemon (*Citrus limon*)
bergamot (*Citrus bergamia*)
rose otto (*Rosa damascena*)

Things to make for your first-aid cabinet

Anti-infectious air spray

For this spray you will need:

120 ml (4 ounces) water
60 ml (2 ounces) alcohol (e.g., vodka)
thyme linalol – 20 drops
cinnamon – 5 drops

clove – 5 drops
tea tree – 10 drops
lemon – 10 drops.

Put the essential oils into the alcohol, then add that to the water and leave it to stand for 24 hours before using. Transfer to a new plant-mister, and spray into the air. Avoid letting the droplets fall on any polished wooden surfaces, delicate materials or other materials, as these could be damaged by the water or other ingredients.

First-aid washing mix

Put the following into a small dropper bottle:

lavender – 30 drops
tea tree – 30 drops
ravensara – 5 drops
eucalyptus radiata – 5 drops
bergamot – 20 drops.

Use 2–6 drops of the mix in a small bowl of water – to wash cuts and grazes. Do not apply neat to any open cut or graze.

Antiseptic skin spray

For this spray you will need:

60 ml (2 ounces) spring water – pre-boiled
15 ml ($\frac{1}{2}$ ounce) alcohol (e.g., vodka)
lavender – 5 drops
tea tree – 10 drops
thyme linalol – 10 drops
chamomile german – 5 drops.

In a clean bottle, combine the essential oils with the alcohol, and shake as vigorously as you can. Then add half the water, a little at a time, and continue shaking. Store for 48 hours. Add the remaining water, and leave for a further 24 hours, shaking the bottle whenever you remember to do so. Then strain through an unbleached paper coffee-filter, and put in a sterile spray bottle.

Antiseptic anti-fungal powder

First, combine the following. Use a blender; otherwise, this could form into a lumpy mass.

50 g green clay
1 teaspoon of finely powdered thyme herb
1 teaspoon of finely powdered marjoram herb.

When combined, slowly add:

tea tree – 15 drops
manuka – 15 drops
palmarosa – 15 drops.

If the mixture is lumpy, simply let it dry out completely, then crush it into a fine powder again.

Herbal healing infused oils

If you want to try making some of your own preparations instead of buying them, various herbs growing in your garden can be used to make herbal healing infused oils. These can't be used as a substitute for essential oils in any of the condition methods in this book, because the strength and properties are different, but infused oils can be used on their own or as a substitute for vegetable carrier oils. Some of the most useful herbal infusions are:

calendula
St John's wort
lemon balm

comfrey
rosemary
marjoram
lavender
rose
chamomile.

Lavender, rose and chamomile can be usefully included in massage oils for very young children. They can also be used as skin-care preparations.

When making infusions, only use fresh, organically grown flowers or herbal materials, and organically produced, cold-pressed vegetable oils. The oil you use is important, as this is what will be applied to your child's skin. Almond oil, sunflower seed oil, olive oil and sesame oil would be good choices for the infusion method (use almond for sensitive skins and sunflower seed for older children). Although olive and sesame oils have their own strong odours, which are likely to mask the odour of the plant material, the plants' healing properties will remain intact.

Tear the plant material up – never use a metallic object, as it can leach out some of the therapeutic properties of the plant. Put the herbs or plant material in a jar that has been sterilized with boiling water – jam-jars (or bottles) with good screw caps can be used to store your oil. Then cover the plant material with your chosen organic oil, such as almond.

Put the jar in a place that catches a lot of sun – a sunny window ledge is ideal. Shake the mixture as often as you can, to help the healing properties of the herb transfer to the oil. Leave the jar in place for between three and seven days. Then strain the oil, using a piece of fine muslin or an unbleached paper coffee-filter. It can take a long time for the oil to seep through a paper filter, but it is an effective way of catching all the plant residue. If you want an even more potent infused oil, repeat the process, using the same oil with fresh plant material. Keep the oil in the fridge.

Natural ointments and salves

You can make your own ointments and salves from scratch, using beeswax and infused oil. To make a soft ointment, you will need:

60 ml (2 ounces) infused oil (of your choice)
15 g (¹/2 ounce) non-refined beeswax
essential oils.

First, put the beeswax into a bowl that is being gently warmed in the *bain-marie* method, where a small bowl is put into a pan of water in order to keep warm. When the beeswax is melted, pour in the oil, stirring all the time, to create a soft ointment. Lastly, while still stirring, add your chosen essential oils and blend them in well. Put the finished mix into jars while still warm, then put the lid on tightly and leave to cool. Keep in the fridge.

As an alternative, purchase a vegetable-based, non-petroleum ointment, and transfer a little to a small, clean, lidded, pot. To this, add some essential oil. Good choices would be antiseptic and anti-bacterial essential oils.

Antiseptic ointment

Blend the following together well:

15 ml (¹/2 ounce) ointment
thyme linalol – 10 drops
ravensara – 5 drops
lavender – 6 drops.

Chest congestion ointment

Blend the following together well:

15 ml ($^{1}/_{2}$ ounce) ointment
ravensara – 10 drops
eucalyptus radiata – 10 drops
niaouli – 5 drops.

Use a small amount each time, rubbed over the chest and back.

Baby oil

Most baby oils are made from mineral-based products, which form a barrier that prevents dampness reaching baby's skin. It is said that these oils cannot be absorbed by the skin. You may like to try this natural alternative based on jojoba oil, which is a natural wax:

15 ml ($^{1}/_{2}$ ounce) jojoba oil
30 ml (1 ounce) almond oil.

Blend well together, then add:

geranium – 2 drops
petitgrain (or lavender) – 2 drops.

Baby powder

Talcum powder has been shown in some research to be potentially damaging to baby's health, but baby powder can be made from simple ingredients that are a safer alternative. You can choose which essential oil to use, from lavender, geranium or petitgrain. Mix the following together in a blender:

30 ml (1 ounce) arrowroot powder
30 ml (1 ounce) cornflour.

Then add into the blender:

your chosen essential oil – 6 drops.

Leave the mixture to dry, then use it as you would talcum powder.

EIGHT

Healing the Sick Child with Essential Oils

An A–Z of conditions

This chapter is an A–Z of the conditions children experience, and suggests different ways of treating them with essential oils. Some physical ailments are not conditions in themselves so much as symptoms of a condition – like a cough, sore throat, fever, headache, rashes, vomiting, diarrhoea or swollen lymph glands. If your child has one of these, especially if there are no other symptoms, look at the section for that symptom, which should help to find the possible cause.

That is not to say you should put yourself in the position of a qualified medical practitioner, as they are there to help. Get whatever assistance you can, and think of essential oils and aromatherapy as nature's nursemaids, offering up their powerful goodness in the quest to keep our children well.

How to use the A–Z

Signs and symptoms

Under each entry, several symptoms are listed. If your child has the condition, they might have just one of the symptoms on the list, several symptoms, or all of them. These will vary from child to child, depending on the severity of the condition and on how the condition happens to manifest itself in your child – which will in part depend on his or her constitution, immunity and home environment. Remember also to read the sections relating to individual symptoms.

Methods

Read all the instructions in the box if you wish to carry out one of the methods. If using a particular method, refer to Chapter 3 for further information; if blending, refer to Chapter 4.

Essential oils that help

If you can't get hold of the essential oils used in the methods outlined, refer to the 'Essential oils that help' list. This contains some essential oils that can help the symptoms of the condition, rather than the condition itself.

Acne

There are two types of acne in children – newborn and teenage.

Newborn acne

Some babies are born with a facial rash that appears rather red and angry, with small red pimples covering the cheeks and nose. It occurs because certain hormones get passed from the mother while baby is in the womb. It will disappear on its own within time, but aromatherapy can help speed up the process. If possible, get a diagnosis from the paediatrician before leaving the maternity unit.

There are three methods you can use, but in all cases first wash the face by using a tiny pinch of very mild, pure soap, and rinse very thoroughly. To see how to carry out the following methods by preparing hydrolats and teas, please refer to page 18. In all cases, dab the area using pure cotton wool.

The most effective method – use lavender and chamomile hydrolat.

 Using the 'infused waters' method: 1 drop each of lavender and chamomile roman essential oils, in $^1/_2$ pint of water.

Put 1 drop of lavender essential oil on an unused chamomile teabag, let it soak in, then allow to dry. When needed, put the teabag in a cup, cover with boiling water and put a saucer on top, so no steam can escape. Allow to cool.

Teenage acne

Acne is really heartbreaking for teenagers, who wish more than anything else to look good to their peers. Acne can affect teenagers emotionally, leading to a loss of self-esteem and self-confidence; also, anxiety and stress are increased, which in turn can make the condition itself worse.

Adolescent or teenage acne is most often caused by increased hormonal activity, which creates an over-production of sebum (the skin's natural moisturizer), and bacteria can flourish in this. Hair follicles as well as pores can become blocked by sebum. In most cases the acne clears up when the hormonal system harmonizes itself in early adulthood, but for many the problem goes on for years. Female adolescents have the added problem that their menstrual cycle can cause acne to erupt every month.

Skin tonics

In equal proportions, mix together pure hydrolats of:

lavender
tea tree
rose.

Pour a small amount of the hydrolat on to cotton wool, and apply gently on the affected areas.

or

Mix the following, and heat gently in a clean pot:

120 ml (4 ounces) rose water
120 ml (4 ounces) aloe vera juice
5 drops lavender
4 drops tea tree.

Leave to cool, then bottle.

Moisturizer

During the day, try to leave the skin exposed to the air as much as possible. Use this moisturizer every evening. Mix the following:

30 ml (1 ounce) jojoba rosemary – 4 drops thyme linalol – 4 drops eucalyptus citriodora – 4 drops

Apply a small amount on the face, then dab off any excess by using a tissue.

Signs and symptoms

 can affect face, neck, back or shoulders

 pimples, whiteheads, blackheads

 infected hair follicles appear reddened, and can cause lumpy cysts to appear under the skin, which themselves can become infected.

Method

Over-the-counter acne preparations may increase the skin's sensitivity. They often leave a fine film on the skin, which can attract more pollution and dirt to it. Stronger formulations for the skin are generally prescribed and sometimes contain antibiotics. These may have side effects. Make sure your child is not using a friend's prescribed medication.

For some unlucky teenagers, acne can have lasting effects in the form of permanent scarring. Encourage your child to take care of their skin by cleaning it as gently as possible, and keeping the skin exposed to fresh air. Cosmetics often cause more problems and may delay the healing process. More importantly, there should be no squeezing or touching of the spots, as this may lead to infection in other areas and can cause scarring and pitting in later life.

This is a disturbed and sensitive time for the skin, as it struggles to find a balance. Whatever the skin type (oily or dry), treat it as gently as possible. Wash with liquid soap (as pure and natural as you can find), rinse off well, then apply one of the tonics, and the moisturizer.

Blackheads

To remove blackheads, first steam the face. Don't squeeze them by hand: use a specialist blackhead remover, or have the job done professionally.

After each one has been removed, dab with a little essential oil of lavender, applied with a cotton-wool bud.

Other spots

Dab some of the following on larger, pus-filled spots. First, put the ingredients in a $1/2$ pint or larger bottle:

$1/4$ bottle dry white wine
camphor – 4 drops
eucalyptus citriodora – 4 drops
lemongrass – 2 drops
thyme linalol – 2 drops
tea tree – 2 drops.

Shake well, and use at least twice a day.

Essential oils that help

lavender
camphor
rosemary
eucalyptus citriodora
tea tree
bergamot
thyme linalol

Arthritis – juvenile rheumatoid

Juvenile rheumatoid arthritis can affect children from as young as two, right through to the teenage years. It's an auto-immune disease, which means the body's immune or defence system attacks the body's own tissues instead of the more usual enemy – invading micro-organisms and other intruders. Depending on the type, rheumatoid arthritis causes inflammation of the joints or internal organs. There are three types:

pauciarticular – less than four areas are affected, such as the knees, elbows or ankles

 polyarticular – when more than five areas or joints are affected, such as fingers, toes, hands and feet

 systematic – when both the joints and internal organs are affected.

The cause of juvenile rheumatoid arthritis is as yet not totally understood. Individual cases can vary, and may be caused by infection, genetic factors or by damage to a joint.

Signs and symptoms

 stiffness in the joints

deformity of the joints caused by tightening of the tendons

swelling, pain and (during later stages of an attack) some skin redness in the area

symptoms can flare up and then go away

Method

Aromatherapy should be seen as a complement to orthodox medical treatment, something in addition to it. The following methods may help ease the pain and stiffness.

Never massage joints or other inflamed parts of the body. If using oils on painful areas, simply apply gently to the skin.

Essential oils that help

lavender
rosemary

57

chamomile roman
myrtle
chamomile german
thyme linalol
eucalyptus radiata
basil linalol
eucalyptus citriodora
marjoram
geranium
ginger

For cold and stiff joints	Inflammation bath blend	Compress method
The following mix can be applied to the joints every day. It can also be applied to joints before getting into a warm bath. Use only a small amount on painful areas.	Apply a small amount to each inflamed area, before getting in a warm bath.	Make up the blend as in 'Inflammation bath blend'. Gently put a small amount on each affected joint, using amounts according to your child's age then cover the area with a cold or warm compress – your child will tell you which is the most comfortable.
First mix together	First, mix together	
ginger – 5 drops marjoram – 5 drops myrtle – 5 drops clove – 2 drops helichrysum – 4 drops.	chamomile german – 10 drops chamomile roman – 5 drops lavender – 10 drops eucalyptus citriodora – 10 drops.	
Then add the appropriate number of drops for your child's age to 30 ml (1 ounce) sesame oil and mix together.	Then add the appropriate number of drops for your child's age to 30 ml (1 ounce) almond oil and mix together.	

Other care

Warmth often helps. For joints that feel painful, cold and very stiff, hold a covered hot-water bottle over the area. For joints that are inflamed and hot to the touch, use a cold compress over the area. The herbal supplement 'cat's claw' can be very helpful, as can 'Devil's claw' (*harpogophylum*). Regular swimming in warm water can help to keep joints supple, as can other forms of gentle exercise.

When to get help

Consult your doctor if any of the following occur:

 The child has a high fever with pain and swelling in the joints or limbs. (Consult immediately.)

 The child has been injured, the injury continues to be painful and sore, and appears red or inflamed.

 The child appears to be limping or not using his or her joints properly.

 Morning stiffness, or if there are general aches and pain around the body.

Asthma

Asthma is caused by irritation in the breathing pathways to the lungs. They become clogged with mucus and constricted, so that inhalation is difficult. Asthma can affect a person at any age, even babies. The attacks range in severity from very mild to life-threatening. Some children stop having attacks around puberty. Asthma often runs in families, and more often occurs in families where there is a history of eczema, psoriasis or hay fever.

There are many 'triggers' to asthma attacks, and they differ from person to person. An attack might be brought on by an ear, nose or throat infection, pollution in the atmosphere, house dust, pets, perfumes and other commercial fragrance products. Some children may have allergies to medications or particular foods – or be sensitive to the preservatives or pesticides used in their manufacture, including sulphates. Stress or anxiety are other factors that might be causing difficulties in breathing.

It's really worthwhile trying to establish which things might 'trigger' your child's asthma attacks. Keep a diary, recording when your child has an attack, noting all the things that happened at the time – what drink or foods were eaten, whether any medication was taken (both for the asthma and for other conditions), whether the child was inside or outside when the attack occurred, pollen conditions, pollution levels, emotional stress, anything surrounding the incident. Ask yourself: 'Did I spray an air freshener or perfume before the attack?' As time goes on and you build up a long-term record, you may be able to identify your child's personal 'triggers', if there are any.

Modern farming methods involve the addition of products that may cause an attack. The growth hormone given to cows, which has been found in some milk, may cause a reaction in some children. Dairy produce also causes the build-up of mucus, so try to cut down on that wherever possible. Wheat and other grains can be a trigger for asthma, especially if grown using pesticides, herbicides or fungicides. Change to organic produce and see if that makes a difference. If not, cut wheat out of the diet altogether for a short period, to see if there is any change. Go through all of the grains in this way, one after the other, and see if there is one that acts as a trigger. Also, cut down on fizzy drinks.

Although pets are a delightful addition to a home, it is possible your child may be allergic to them. Compare your child's incidence of attacks when around animals and when away from them. Also, be aware of your own moods. Many children take on the emotions of their parents/carers, so if you feel anxious the child may do so too, and may have an attack because of it. Let your child be a child, unburdened by worries for as long as you can, but don't mollycoddle. Allow him or her to run free and exercise, if well enough to do so.

Signs and symptoms

  wheezing with coughing

  coughing when trying to exhale; difficulty exhaling breath

  pains in the chest when breathing

  a feeling of constriction or tightness in the chest

Method

The very fact of having an asthma attack can cause a child to feel anxious. The following mixture of essential oils may help to calm your child, thus allowing peaceful sleep. Also, having this calming bath before bed may prevent an anxiety-induced attack during the night.

Bath mix – to calm

First, mix the following essential oils in 30 ml (1 ounce) vegetable oil:

chamomile roman – 5 drops
mandarin – 4 drops
geranium – 1 drop.

Then add the following amount to a bath, according to the age of the child:

up to 4 – $1/4$ teaspoon
5–8 years – $1/2$ teaspoon
8–12 years – 1 teaspoon.

Back massage may help to reduce the incidence of asthma attacks. Massage over the whole of the back in large, sweeping movements in an upward direction. Also massage the chest in the same way, more gently this time. Use enough of the massage oil so the area is covered, but not so much that the skin remains greasy. For babies under 2 years of age, don't use the whole teaspoon of mix – just use a tiny amount.

Massage and inhalation mix

First, make up a mix of essential oils, using these proportions:

niaouli – 10 drops
marjoram – 4 drops
frankincense – 2 drops
chamomile roman – 10 drops.

Bottle the mix for future use.

Essential oils that help

lavender
marjoram
geranium
petitgrain
frankincense
chamomile german
cypress
chamomile roman
niaouli

Inhalation

One drop of the mix can be put on a tissue and inhaled when the child feels an attack may be coming, or if the child is under stress and you think he or she may have an attack.

Back and chest massage

To make a massage oil, take the following number of drops from the bottle, depending on the age of the child, and dilute in 5ml to 10ml of vegetable oil.

up to 2 years – 1 drop (use only a tiny amount each time)
2–5 years – 2 drops
6–8 years – 3 drops
9–11 years – 4 drops
12–16 years – 5 drops

Other care

Buteyko is a breathing technique developed by a Russian doctor, and has been shown to be helpful in cutting down the incidence of asthma attacks. Search the internet for 'buteyko', or see if your local bookshop has anything on the subject.

Encourage your child to follow the Cave Man Eating Plan (see page 24).

Alternative massage mixes

Under 2 years
Mix in 30 ml (I ounce) vegetable oil:
lavender – 3 drops

OR

geranium – 2 drops.

2–7 year olds
Mix in 30 ml (I ounce) vegetable oil:
3 drops lavender
2 drops geranium
I drop frankincense.

Over 7 years
Mix in 30 ml (I ounce) vegetable oil:
geranium – 2 drops
cypress – 2 drops
frankincense – 2 drops.

When to get help

Get immediate medical attention if your child does not respond to his or her regular medication.

PREVENTION

   Keep a diary of possible 'triggers'.

   Let the child exercise.

   Try not to let the child be aware of your own stress.

Athlete's foot

This fungal infection is called 'athlete's foot' because it is often picked up by sporty types, who spend a lot of time walking around communal changing rooms, showers or swimming pools. It can also be transmitted by sharing footwear, towels and bathmats. It's caused by the fungus *tinea*, and affects the toenails, the soles of the feet and the area between the toes.

Signs and symptoms

   soft, white, scaling skin; dry, peeling skin; cracking, open flesh

   itching between the toes; burning sensation; redness

   thickened, yellowing toenails

   foot odour

   possibly a rash resembling a group of small blisters

Method

Footbath and dab

Prepare the footbath in an old plastic washing-up bowl, or something similar.

Fill with warm water and add:

1 tablespoon bicarbonate of soda
1 tablespoon Epsom salts
2 tablespoons cider vinegar
tea tree – 5 drops.

Soak the feet for at least five minutes a day, and dry them thoroughly. Then, using a cotton-wool bud, dab between the toes and around the toenails with this concentrated essential oil mix (using only a tiny dab each time):

tea tree – 30 drops   cypress – 2 drops.
manuka – 30 drops

If your child catches athlete's foot, the feet should be kept as clean and dry as possible, and bathing them several times a day does help with the itching. This is obviously difficult to manage when the child is at school all day, so just do what you can.

Foot powder	Foot massage oil
Powder between the toes every day with a small amount of the following:	Apply to the affected areas. Use a small amount of the following each time:
100 g green clay tea tree – 10 drops manuka – 10 drops.	1 tablespoon sesame oil tea tree – 5 drops lemon – 1 drop manuka – 3 drops.
Mix the ingredients in a blender. Alternatively, just add the essential oils to the clay, while stirring fast. It will still go lumpy, so wait for it to dry, then crunch the lumps into the rest of the clay and mix well.	This is easiest to use at night, after the footbath, and having dried the feet well.

Essential oils that help

Some essential oils are appropriate for adult use, but with children only the following are recommended:

tea tree
cypress
manuka
palmarosa
lemongrass.

When to get help

If the fungus appears to be spreading, seek professional advice.

If there is no improvement after three weeks of either pharmaceutical or home-help treatment, seek further professional advice.

PREVENTION

 This fungus likes damp skin, so always dry feet thoroughly and try to keep feet out of trainers for at least some of the time. Don't let your child go barefoot, but he or she can wear open-toed shoes around the house, or sandals if the weather is fine.

 Choose natural-fibre socks – preferably cotton. Use clean socks each day.

 Make sure shoes are thoroughly dry before using.

 Use anti-fungal preparations in both shoes after each wear, especially if other members of the household also have athlete's foot.

Attention Deficit Disorder (ADD)

A huge number of children are being diagnosed as having an attention deficit disorder, and many are on medication for it. ADD covers a wide range of characteristic behaviour patterns relating to learning capacity and social skills. As a society, we should be concerned that so many of our children are experiencing these difficulties.

Figures show that ADD affects more boys than girls, and seems to run in families. Attention deficit disorders (ADD) include a condition known as ADHD – attention deficit hyperactive disorder – additional help for this can be found on page 70. Children under three years of age cannot be diagnosed as having ADD or ADHD, or put on medication for it, because the symptoms of the disorder could be said to apply to all normal children of this age.

Signs and symptoms

   poor attention span; easily distracted; difficulty in concentration

   disorganized and losing things frequently; learning disorders

   difficulty following instructions; difficulty in accepting authority

   impulsive behaviour; mood swings

   poor school performance

   ADHD – hyperactivity; sleeplessness; headaches

There are also other quite specific symptom indicators, such as shouting out the answer in class before being asked by the teacher, being disruptive in class, and not being able to wait or queue patiently. Children can also engage in dangerous behaviour, almost as if they have lost their sense of fear. This is what worries society so greatly – children out of control – and it perhaps explains why so many children are put on medication.

At present, there is no known specific cause of ADD, and it's likely there are many factors involved. Symptoms vary from child to child, and some may have developed the condition because of a nervous system disorder, dysfunctional brain development, brain injury, or having been born premature or a drug-dependent baby. Other causes of ADD may be environmental, such as chemical farming methods and food additives, or industrial and vehicle pollution. It has even been suggested that ADD is caused by immunization.

Before worrying about all these things, we need first to ask if the child actually has an attention deficit disorder. The symptoms listed above could be applied to many children who are going through the normal development process. All children get bored and frustrated, and act impulsively. One symptom of ADD is given as 'not being able to play with one toy, but moving on to another'. All children do this, and if some do it faster than others it is not surprising, given the type of society we live in. Think about the television – with so many channels to choose from, we flick between them rapidly with our remote controls. Children grow up with this, so it's not surprising if they think it's normal to change from one toy to another, just as we flick between channels. If we want our children to concentrate on one thing at a time, we have to give them an environment in which they can learn such a skill, or spend time with them, teaching them how to do so. There was a time when children spent hours pushing the same car around the floor; now they have computers and zap monsters at double-quick time.

Other characteristics of ADD could equally be applied to adults – making careless mistakes, not paying close attention to instructions, disrespect of authority, not finishing assignments because there is something else to do. Our children do not live in a vacuum – they watch and copy us.

For whatever reason, however, some children do have what might be diagnosed as ADD, and essential oils may be able to help calm them.

Method

Soothing baths and showers

All children have to wash, and essential oils can help make this a time of calming down and soothing. First, in a small bottle, mix the essential oils together in these proportions:

mandarin – 20 drops
lavender – 10 drops
chamomile roman –
10 drops.

Baths

Dilute the essential oil mix in 1 teaspoon vegetable oil, using these amounts:

3–5 years – 2 drops
6–8 years – 3 drops
8–11 years – 5 drops.

Add to the bath water, and swish around before the child gets in.

Showers

Before taking a shower, after the right water temperature has been reached, put 4 drops of the essential oil mix on a facecloth or sponge, and place it at the bottom of the shower cubicle.

Body oil

You can apply the body oil on younger children, but older children will probably want to apply body oil themselves – although getting them to remember to do it might be difficult! Use a small amount each time; massaging on the back is best for this disorder.

Dilute the appropriate number of drops for your child's age from the following mix, adding the essential oils to 30 ml (1 ounce) vegetable oil:

tangerine – 10 drops
cardamom – 5 drops
lavender – 5 drops.

Helping concentration

Studies have shown that essential oils can help with focus and concentration. Diffuse essential oils in the atmosphere, such as:

lemon
bergamot
grapefruit
pine.

Helping sleep

Studies have also shown that sleep can be easier when essential oils are used. Lavender would be an excellent choice. Diffuse it in the room before going to bed (but not overnight). Or place a drop of lavender oil on the underside of the pillow, away from the eyes – it doesn't stain, and washes out easily. A child with ADD will need 1–2 drops, but if the child is on medication use only 1 drop.

Essential oils that help

The following essential oils are easily available and they help to soothe and calm children of all ages:

mandarin
petitgrain
tangerine
ho wood
chamomile roman
lavender.

Other care

Certain components in food are thought to make hyperactivity worse. Try to persuade your child to follow the Cave Man Eating Plan (see page 24), or at least cut down on the caffeine in fizzy drinks, sugar in general, and processed foods. Avoid food colourings wherever you can.

Find time to talk to your child, and play together. Younger children can be discouraged from spending time watching TV and sitting in front of the computer. See also *Computer-related problems.*

When to get help

Correct diagnosis is very important, and before medication is given you should get a second professional opinion. Your child may just be at a hyperactive stage of development. The symptoms of ADD may also be an expression of your child's frustration at having an undiagnosed learning difficulty, such as dyslexia. Try to remember that most children go through a stage of hyperactivity at some time in their lives, sometimes only briefly. Above all, ensure that your child is not just seeking your attention because they feel they have too little of it. Time spent with a child reading, playing outside games or indoor board games and so on pays great dividends in terms of good behaviour.

PREVENTION

 Assess your child for learning difficulty.

 Change your child's diet.

 Do activities with child.

 Create a soothing atmosphere in the home.

Balanitis

Balanitis is inflammation of the penis head (the glans). It can be caused by several things, including bacteria, fungi, wearing tight clothes or having an allergy to the chemicals in nappies or clothes. It can also be caused by nappy rash. Balanitis is more likely in uncircumcized boys.

Signs and symptoms

 inflamed and sore penis – on the tip, or under and around the foreskin

 (if the child is in nappies) infected buttocks and genital area

 swollen penis

 difficulty in drawing back the foreskin for cleaning

Method

Bathing

Essential oils in the bath ease irritation and discomfort. Use half this amount when the child is between 5 and 10 years old, and all if the child is older. Mix together:

1 teaspoon vegetable oil
chamomile german – 3 drops
tea tree – 2 drops
palmarosa – 1 drop.

Ointment

Apply a small amount of the ointment, and apply as needed.

15 ml (¹/₂ ounce) aloe vera gel
15 ml (¹/₂ ounce) calendula-infused oil
jojoba – 10 drops
lavender – 6 drops
geranium – 4 drops.

Essential oils that help

lavender   thyme linalol
manuka   tea tree
chamomile german   palmarosa

Babies up to 2 years

Follow directions for **Nappy rash** (see page 219).

Other care

Ensure the child bathes regularly, drawing back the foreskin gently to clean the area. Dry the penis thoroughly after every nappy change, or tell older children to dry themselves. Then apply the ointment.

If you suspect your washing powder has caused an allergic reaction in your child, rinse and dry clothes already laundered, and change your washing powder with the next wash.

When to get help

If an infection appears, or there is pus coming from the penis, tell your doctor. If the condition does not improve after a few days of home treatment – natural or pharmaceutical – go for further help.

PREVENTION

 Ensure there is good hygiene.

 Check that washing products are not causing an allergic reaction.

 Make sure your child's pants or nappy is not too tight.

Bites – animal and insect

Children come into contact with all kinds of animals, both domestic and wild. Animal bites can be extremely dangerous and should always be seen by a doctor or hospital as soon as possible. A tetanus injection may be needed if your child's inoculation has not been kept up-to-date. This section offers immediate self-help advice on animal, snake and insect bites, which you can carry out while waiting for further professional help.

Method

Animals

Wash the area of the bite with water and mild soap, and then with water and disinfectant. If the area is easily accessible, rinse in water running gently from a tap, for several minutes. Then dry and cover. If the wound is bleeding, apply pressure to the area with a clean piece of material, and make sure further help for the child is being arranged.

Rabies is a worry, especially where wildlife is concerned, although superficial wounds are not as risky as those that puncture the skin. If the skin is broken at all, or there is bleeding, or more than one bite, call your doctor immediately. Even if the skin was not broken at the time, if it starts to look red and swollen later or infected under the surface, get immediate medical help.

Snake bites

Try to keep both the child and yourself calm, and arrange for emergency medical help immediately. The bitten area should be kept as still as possible, so try to avoid unnecessary movement. While getting help, cover the bite with a cold compress, on which you have put at least 25 drops of lavender oil. If you don't have any lavender to hand, use what you have – any essential oil is better than none at this point.

It's difficult to know whether the bite is poisonous or not, so just err on the side of caution and assume it is. It's highly likely the bite was poisonous if the fang marks are deep and prominent, or if any of the following symptoms occur:

  swelling, redness, bluishness, or a burning sensation around the area of the bite

  the tissue around the bite, as well as the bite area itself, is very painful

  feeling faint, nausea, vomiting

  clammy skin; sweating

  rapid, too shallow breathing

  fast heart and pulse rate.

Insect bites

Insect bites cause pain, soreness, itching, swelling and redness. Whatever the insect, get help if the child develops a rash or if the bite looks infected. If the child has difficulty in breathing, get help quickly.

Allergic reaction to insect bites is common, and signs may appear over the following 12 – 24 hours. Look for increased swelling in the area, redness or hives. If any of these occur, or if the child is in pain, has breathing difficulties, nausea or headache, get immediate medical attention.

Most insect bites can be soothed by applying a cold, wet compress, on which 5 drops each of chamomile german and lavender have been put. For more specific information, see below:

Spiders

Mix the following together and apply a small amount to the area three times over the next 24 hours, or longer if needed:

1 teaspoon alcohol
3 drops lavender
2 drops chamomile german.

The black-widow spider bite is particularly nasty, and is one of those that requires immediate attention. On your way to getting medical help, apply 10 drops of neat lavender oil directly on to the bite every five minutes, until you arrive.

Mosquitoes

Prevention is best where mosquitoes are concerned, and they are deterred from coming too close by the smell of lavender. Put drops of neat lavender oil on clothing – on socks, cloth shoes, collars, sleeves, and the bottom of skirts or trouser legs, making sure the drops are not next to the skin. At night, put lavender oil on tissues or cotton wool and tuck under your child's pillow, or put on the bedside table. Other oils that help keep mosquitoes away are lemongrass, citronella and eucalyptus citriodora.

For single bites:

put 1 drop of neat lavender oil directly on the bite.

For multiple bites, mix:

250 ml (8 ounces) cider vinegar (or the juice of 2 lemons)
lavender – 10 drops
thyme linalol – 5 drops.

Put the mixture in the bath, swishing the water around before putting the child in. Afterwards, put neat lavender on the bites.

Gnat and midge bites	Bee stings	Wasp or bee stings
To stop the irritation, mix the following and apply over the whole affected area:	Bee stings can cause fever and headaches, and if there's an allergic reaction there can be swelling, redness and a rash and medical attention is required. Try to remove the sting. Put a few drops of chamomile german on a cold cider-vinegar compress and apply to the area. If the position of the bite allows, leave the compress there for a couple of hours; otherwise, for as long as possible. Then apply 1 drop of neat chamomile german to the bite, three times a day for two days.	Mix the following and dab on to the bitten area, three times a day:
1 teaspoon cider vinegar (or lemon juice)		1 teaspoon cider (or wine) vinegar
thyme linalol – 3 drops		lavender – 2 drops.
1 tablespoon lavender hydrolat (or plain water).		
Alternatively, apply neat lavender oil to the bites.		

Essential oils that help

thyme
chamomile german
oregano
manuka
eucalyptus radiata

lemongrass
ravensara
geranium
lavender

Blisters

Although the most common type of blister is the one caused by a shoe rubbing on the skin, there are other, more worrying varieties. Blisters can form anywhere on the body due to an allergy, or viral or bacterial infection. For blisters caused by burns, see *Burns* and *Sunburn* (pages 92 and 261).

Signs and symptoms

 raised, thin skin filled with fluid, surrounding redness; sore if pressed

Method

Blisters on the feet

Blisters form as a way of protection – to stop further damage to the tissue. They generally clear up by themselves over time. See 'Other care' below.

If the skin is not broken, apply a drop of neat lavender or lemon essential oil.

Recycle those old teabags! Put 1 drop of geranium on a wet teabag (black or green tea), and hold it over the blister.

If your child plays a lot of sports, or is always wearing trainers and has repeated trouble with blisters, it may be worth toughening up his or her feet. Mix the following together well, and soak the feet for 10 minutes at least once a week:

a bowl of cold tea
1 tablespoon Epsom salts
1 drop of myrrh essential oil diluted in 1 drop iodine.

Blisters on the body

Blisters on the body are a sign of infection or other problem that requires medical help. In the meantime, to help reduce the inflammation and pain, make up the hydrolat mix below, put in a new plant mister, and spray over the affected area (see page 18 for how to make a hydrolat).

equal parts of lavender, chamomile and rose hydrolat
chamomile roman – 3 drops
eucalyptus radiata – 3 drops

Shake well before use.

Essential oils that help

tea tree
lavender
lemon
chamomile roman
calendula (infused or absolute)

Other care

Always leave the blister as it is, and never try to get the fluid out while the skin underneath is in the process of healing. Leave the blistered area uncovered as much as possible so it has a chance to dry out and heal.

When to get help

Always consult a doctor if there are blisters on the body, if the child has a fever, or has blisters due to an allergy or as a result of taking medication. Also, get further help if the blisters become infected or have increased redness around the outer edges, or if there is swelling.

PREVENTION

   Wear well-fitting shoes.

   Wear socks with trainers.

   At the first sign of redness, protect heels or sore patches of the foot with blister dressings.

Body-piercing

Body-piercing appeals even to young children, who often find that a professional body-piercer will not carry out the work on them without their parents' consent. Consequently, children sometimes attempt to carry out their own body-piercing, or do it for their friends. However it is carried out, body-piercing often results in soreness, infection and inflammation.

The area is infected if it is red, swollen, feels raw and/or there is a discharge. This discharge often dries into a crust around the ring or other pierced object, and in the immediate body area affected. If this occurs, the pierced object should be removed – earrings can be removed easily, but any other body-piercing should be removed professionally.

Infection arises when bacteria get into the wounded area, and it's vital that it is kept clean at all times. Pierced ears are at risk of infection from nearby hair, touching by fingers, and from bedlinen. If the piercing is covered by clothing, keep it covered with a sterile dressing. Otherwise, expose the area as much as possible because light and air assist in the healing process. Body-piercings are prone to repeat infections, which can cause scar tissue under the surface of the skin and scarring on the surface.

Method

Immediate Preventative Care

Prevention is best. So if your child has just had a body-piercing, to help prevent infection get a bowl of water and add 2 tablespoons of salt and 1 drop of tea tree oil to each pint of water. Bathe the pierced area with this salted water.

Sore holes

Add these essential oils to 8 ml (¼ ounce) alcohol:
tea tree – 5 drops
geranium – 5 drops.

Add all this to a bowl of salt-water and bathe the affected area(s).

Infected holes (anywhere on the body)

First, remove the pierced object. Clean the area at least four times a day with the alcohol mix on the left under 'Sore holes'.

Then, use 1 drop of the following mix of essential oils over the affected area:

thyme linalol – 8 drops
ravensara – 5 drops
lavender – 6 drops
tea tree – 7 drops.

Do not use on mucous membrane areas.

In the mouth (anywhere on the body)

Rinse the mouth out at least five times a day with the following, then spit it out. Add these essential oils to 30 ml (1 ounce) alcohol:

myrrh – 10 drops
frankincense – 2 drops
clove – 3 drops.

Blend together well, then bottle up. Use 10 drops of this mix, added to a small glass of salted water, for each mouth rinse.

Essential oils that help

thyme linalol
frankincense
clove
ravensara
tea tree
niaouli
myrrh
(Lavender may assist in closing the hole.)

Other care

Tincture of myrrh – for mouth or tongue-piercings only.

Boils

A boil is a skin infection, usually caused by *staphylococcus* bacteria. The boil forms into a pus-filled lumpy area under the surface of the skin, and is very sore and painful. However, it shouldn't be confused with a pus-filled spot, which is near the surface of the skin (see *Acne*). Children of all ages can develop boils, whether they are babies or teenagers. Boils can appear on all areas, particularly the buttocks, face, nose, neck, ears, back, armpits and groin. An infected hair follicle can often result in a boil.

Signs and symptoms

 a sore and painful red lump under the surface of the skin, which becomes harder over time

 occasionally, soreness around the affected area

 often, swollen lymph glands

Method

Washing	Hot compresses and oil method
Bathe the area twice a day with the following essential oils, which have been put in a small bowl of hot water and swished around:	To draw out the pus, put 1 drop of thyme linalol on a hot compress. Apply afresh twice a day.
lavender – 2 drops tea tree – 2 drops.	When the pus has come out, apply a small amount of the following mix around the area, again twice a day:
If the inflammation is severe, add:	lavender – 3 drops tea tree – 2 drops.
chamomile – 1 drop.	

While pus is coming out of the boil, it's extremely important to keep the area as clean as possible and change dressings frequently. Be careful that no pus gets on any other part of the body, as this may cause further infection and boils. Epsom salts and sea salt are effective additions to water when cleansing the area. If the boil is on the buttocks, find a bowl large enough for the child to be able to sit in. Fill the bowl with warm water and add 1 tablespoon of salt. Then ask your child to sit in it for a few minutes.

While pus is coming out

Cleansing soak

The following mix can be used to soak the area of the boil. If the area cannot be soaked, use the mix to wash the area as often as possible. Swish around to disperse oils before use.

2 pints water
I teaspoon Epsom salts
I teaspoon sea salt
lavender – 2 drops
tea tree – 2 drops
thyme linalol – I drop.

Larger quantities can be made, using the same proportions.

Compresses

To draw out the pus – make the cleansing soak mix (see left) using boiling water, then soak a clean piece of lightweight natural material in it (muslin is ideal), squeeze out and hold over the boil until cool. Repeat three times.

Then, cover the boil with a dressing on which you've put I drop lemon oil and I drop lavender oil and left to dry. The part of the dressing with the essential oils on should be directly over the boil.

Essential oils that help

lavender
tea tree
manuka
lemon
thyme linalol
eucalyptus radiata

Other care

Treat boils as an infection and do not share towels, facecloths, etc. Do not squeeze boils – they will eventually come to a head and burst. Keep the area covered to prevent further infection, and change dressings frequently. If the boil is on an area that gets rubbed by clothes, apply an extra-large, thick dressing to make it less sore. If the boil is on a baby's buttocks, change nappies more frequently and, whenever possible, expose the skin to the air.

When to get help

It is vital that you get immediate medical help if you notice a thin red line running away from the boil to the neck, armpit or groin. This line may be a sign that the infection is spreading through the bloodstream to other areas of the body.

Continuously getting boils may indicate there is another disorder present, so a doctor's advice should be sought. Also contact your doctor if there is more than one boil and they seem to be multiplying, if your child feels ill/has a fever, or if the infection does not clear up after the boil has discharged all the pus. Boils sometimes need to be lanced. You should never do this yourself – always get a qualified medical practitioner to carry this out.

PREVENTION

 Keep body-hair areas scrupulously clean. Sometimes, if clothes have been rubbing against the skin, bacteria enter the hair follicle and boils start to appear.

Broken bones – fractures

Bones can be broken, splintered, displaced or dislocated at the joint, and the only way to know the exact nature of the damage is to get an X-ray and immediate medical attention. Hairline fractures in small children may only need to be in plaster for a few days. Children's bones are more pliable than adults', and sometimes bend rather than break.

Although a broken bone needs to be set in plaster as soon as possible, home help can help the mind and body to cope with the trauma, so that all the body's healing energy is focused on repairing the fracture as quickly as possible.

Signs and symptoms

 pain

 swelling

 lack of mobility

Method

To ease the trauma

To help with the pain and to calm the child, put a few drops of lavender essential oil near the break, and spread it very gently around.

To help speed healing

After the bone has been set in plaster, essential oils can be put on the exposed surrounding skin. Take care not to move or dislodge the bone. Simply smooth the mix on the available skin; do not massage or rub it in. The following mix can be used on children over 5 years of age. Use a small amount only with each application:

8 ml (¹/₄ ounce) St John's Wort-infused oil
ginger – 10 drops
lavender – 5 drops
helichrysum – 2 drops.

Essential oils that help

lavender
myrtle
ginger
spikenard
chamomile roman
helichrysum
St John's Wort-infused oil
calendula-infused oil

Other care

Cold compresses may help ease the pain while you are waiting for medical help. These can be made using cold water, or witch hazel, or a solution of water and the essential oils listed above. Homeopathic arnica tablets can also be given, as well as Dr Bach's Rescue Remedy – both are available in most large chemists and in health-food shops.

When to get help

Always get emergency medical help immediately.

Bronchiolitis

For children over 2 years of age, *see also Bronchitis.*

Bronchiolitis is an infection of the bronchioles (air tubes), and mostly affects babies and children under 2 years of age. The infection is usually viral, such as respiratory syncytial virus, among others, and results in inflammation and narrowing of the air tubes, along with a build-up of mucus.

The infection is easily spread in the air, and can even contaminate surfaces, which are then touched by the young child. As it's more usual in the colder months, the first symptoms are often mistaken for the common cold. Antibiotics are not usually effective against this type of virus, while essential oils can be highly useful.

Keep your baby warm, cosy and calm by paying him or her lots of attention. Give plenty of liquids, and feed baby small amounts frequently, rather than large amounts infrequently.

Signs and symptoms

   runny nose, sniffles, sneezing, coughing

   rapid breathing, shallow breaths, wheezing, inability to breathe properly

   temperature, fever, feeling generally unwell

   refusal of food and fluids

   sometimes, bluish lips and mouth

   possibility of being mistaken for the common cold

Method

Bronchiolitis mix

The following mix can be used in three ways. Make up an amount, using these proportions, then bottle it:

niaouli – 20 drops
ravensara – 10 drops
thyme linalol – 8 drops.

Room steamer

Put the essential oils into a bowl of steaming-hot water and place in the same room as baby, out of reach of children and pets. Use these amounts, according to the age of the baby:

under 1 year – 5 drops
over 1 year – 8 drops.

Drops on material

To help breathing during the night, put 2 drops of the mix on the back of your child's nightclothes, and on a corner of a pillow or mattress cover. Always place drops somewhere away from the eyes.

Massage

Use 5 drops of the above mix in 1 teaspoon almond oil.

With children under 2 years of age, rub a small amount of this over the back of the body. Imagine where the lungs are, then apply on that area of the child's back. Do this twice a day.

For children over 2 years old, before applying the oil put 2 drops of the mix directly on your hands, rub them together and wipe over the child's front and back. Then apply a small amount of the massage oil over the back, as above.

Essential oils that help fight the infection *Suitable for young children*	Essential oils that help keep the child calm *Suitable for young children*
niaouli ravensara eucalyptus radiata thyme linalol myrtle	lavender chamomile roman mandarin *Can be diluted and massaged into the feet.*

Other care

Give your child plenty of fluids to drink. To prevent him or her becoming distressed (which makes breathing more difficult), soothe your child. The British Medical Association recommends using steam such as a humidifier, or steam from a bowl. Keep it well out of the reach of the child, to avoid burns.

When to get help

As soon as your child develops cold-like symptoms, keep a close eye on him or her to make sure the infection does not worsen. If it does, seek medical attention, as the child may need oxygen to enable proper breathing. Hospitalization may be required.

PREVENTION

 Keep babies and young children away from anyone who is sneezing, or shows signs of having a cold or flu.

 If someone living in the home has a cold or flu, diffuse essential oils throughout the house to help keep it from being passed on (see the list of oils for fighting infection above).

If someone travelling in the same car as the baby has a cold or flu, put 1 drop of essential oil (from the 'fighting infection' list above) on a tissue and tuck it near baby's seat (though out of reach).

Bronchitis

Bronchitis is an inflammation of the membranes lining the airways (bronchial tubes). It is usually a complication of a viral or bacterial infection, which often starts with cold- or flu-type symptoms – runny nose, sniffles, sore throat, developing into a deep, chesty cough. The inflammation can be made worse by a smoky or polluted atmosphere.

Keep the child as calm and distress-free as possible. It's better that the phlegm is released rather then held in, so try to get the child to spit out any phlegm. See 'Other care' below.

Signs and symptoms

  dry cough or mucous cough, which feels sore when child coughs

  yellow phlegm

  wheezing; chest pain

  fever

Method

Bronchitis mix

The following mix can be used in three ways. Make up an amount, using these proportions, and bottle:

thyme linalol – 10 drops   niaouli – 10 drops
eucalyptus radiata – 10 drops   myrtle – 25 drops.

Room steamer	*Tissue*	*Massage*
Put 10 drops of the bronchitis mix into a bowl of steaming-hot water and place in the same room as the child – but out reach of them, other children and pets.	To help breathing during the night, put 2 drops on a tissue and tuck near the child's head, away from his or her eyes.	Use 2–4 drops of the above mix in 1 teaspoon vegetable oil, then massage a small amount over the child's chest and back.

Essential oils that help

niaouli
ravensara
myrtle
thyme linalol
eucalyptus radiata
essential oil-prepared blends for breathing, such as Bronchodect (see 'Suppliers', page 313)

Other care

The British Medical Association recommends humidifiers or steam to help keep the bronchial passages clear. Both methods can be used with essential oils. If the child is coughing, to encourage the release of phlegm hold him or her over your lap, front down. Keep the child's head propped up at night. Get him or her to drink plenty of liquid, and to eat frequent, small meals rather than infrequent, large ones.

When to get help

There can be complications with bronchitis, so always get a diagnosis and be prepared to contact help again if the condition gets worse, or if it doesn't seem to be getting better. Get immediate help if the child is wheezing, vomiting or has a bluish tinge around the lips and mouth.

PREVENTION

 Same as for *Bronchiolitis* (see page 86).

Burns

No matter how vigilant we are, children get themselves into accidents. That is simply their nature, as they like to explore and move about, and sometimes they will get burned. Children are burned not only by fire, but also by hot objects, hot liquids, steam, electricity, radiation and chemicals. Electrical burns are often worse than they look, so get an immediate medical opinion on them. Shock is a danger with all burns, and it may come on hours after the event. It's always better to be on the safe side, so get a professional opinion.

Signs and symptoms

 First-degree or superficial burns
There is a red area or patch of skin, over which a blister might form, filled with a water-like substance. Only small burns of this type can be treated with the following suggestions.

 Second-degree burns
There is a great deal of pain, redness, swelling or blistering. Immediate emergency medical treatment must be sought.

 Third-degree burns
These burns affect the deeper tissue of the body and are very dangerous. The skin may appear brown or black instead of red, and because the nerve endings are damaged there may be no pain. Immediate emergency medical treatment must be sought.

Method

First action – all burns

Cool the skin by immersing in cold water – the colder, the better, but do not use ice directly on the skin. This water can be from a sink or bath tap or a shower – whatever source is nearest. Adjust the tap until the water is flowing gently, put the burned area into the flow, and keep the child as still as possible until the area cools down (10 minutes or so).

You could also use cold water in a bowl, and add a couple of ice cubes to keep it cool. If the skin is intact, add a few drops of lavender oil to the cold water and swish it around.

If the burn appears to be anything more than superficial, arrange for medical help immediately .

Second action – home treatment

1 If no broken skin or broken blisters, put 2 drops of neat lavender oil directly on the area of the burn.

2 If the skin is broken or the blister is broken, put 2 drops of neat lavender oil around the area of the burn.

All cases – then put 5 drops of lavender oil on a dry, cold compress, leave to dry and use it to cover the area.

Repeat 1) or 2) (as appropriate) and compress (if needed).

Heat burns

Apply a cold compress.

Chemical burns

Cover the area with a clean dressing. Get to your hospital A&E department immediately if a lower layer of skin has been exposed, or if there are signs of infection, or damage other than redness.

Essential oils that help

lavender
chamomile german

Other care

Cover the burned area with clean, non-fluffy material. Don't apply any greasy substances, such as butter, margarine or vegetable oil. Give the child lots of cool drinks, and keep his or her body warm.

When to get help

Remember that with burns there is a danger of your child going into shock (see *Shock*). Always call your doctor if the burn is from a chemical or electrical source, even if the burn appears only superficial.

In the case of other burns, get medical attention if it does not appear to be healing, if it becomes more red or swollen, or if it develops areas of pus.

PREVENTION

 Keep your child away from fire, matches and cigarettes.

 Check that dangerous chemicals and other liquids are not within reach.

 Check that electrical equipment and wiring is not within reach, and that wall sockets are fitted with child-protection covers.

Catarrh

When a child has too much mucus in the throat and nose, it's called catarrh. It's one of the body's self-defence mechanisms, as it produces mucus to try and rid the body of bacteria, viruses and other irritants. Catarrh usually accompanies or follows conditions that affect the respiratory system, such as colds, flu, hayfever, sinusitis – even measles and ear infections.

Signs and symptoms

 stuffed-up nose; inability to breathe easily

 runny nose

 coughing

Method

Humidifier

Add to the water in the humidifier:

ravensara – 4 drops
eucalyptus radiata – 2 drops.

If the inflammation is severe, add:

chamomile – 1 drop.

Chest rub

The following mix will help clear the congestion in the chest.

Dilute in 1 teaspoon vegetable oil, and apply a small amount on the chest and back, before bedtime:

ravensara – 3 drops
eucalyptus radiata – 1 drop.

Steaming-bowl inhalation method

This method should only be used with children who are old/sensible enough to understand why they should keep their hands off the table and out of the way of the hot water. To a small bowl of steaming water, add:

eucalyptus radiata – 4 drops.

Alternatively, use menthol crystals.

Your child should inhale the aromatic steam through the nose, and the mouth and eyes need to be kept shut. Put a towel over your child's head – big enough to hang down to the shoulders – in order to stop the steam escaping.

Essential oils that help

ravensara
eucalyptus radiata
niaouli
elemi
frankincense

Other care

Breathing at night will be made easier if you prop your child up against pillows. Give him or her child plenty of drinks. Make sure your child's nose is blown and throat cleared, rather than letting him or her sniff the mucus back up.

When to get help

With a baby, get help if the catarrh is making feeding difficult, or if you think baby's catarrh is due to an allergy. Also seek medical advice if your child has an ear infection that is causing the catarrh.

Chickenpox

Chickenpox is a contagious viral infection that can only be caught by being in direct contact with a person who has either chickenpox, or shingles (the adult version of the infection). It's spread very easily from child to child, and although it's said that a child's immunity to it is built up after having it once, the fact is some children have chickenpox two or three times during their childhood years. Chickenpox affects children of all ages.

Children with weakened immune systems can have the disease far more seriously than those who have healthy immune systems. It's important the infected child doesn't scratch the scabs, as that can cause infection, or scarring in later life.

To help prevent other people in the household catching chickenpox, spray the atmosphere with anti-viral essential oils (see Chapters 3 and 7).

Signs and symptoms

 First sign – mild fever, feeling unwell and/or cranky, headache, chills; then

 Second sign – a rash of small red spots on the child's body and scalp – turning to

 Third sign – fluid-filled blisters, that cause intense itching – turning to

 Last sign – scabs, which eventually drop off.

Method

Diffuser mix to aid sleep	Calamine lotion and essential oil mix
To help induce sleep, use the following essential oils in a diffuser or spray:	To a 250 ml (8 ounce) bottle of calamine lotion, add:
lavender – 2 drops petitgrain – 4 drops.	chamomile german – 10 drops lavender – 30 drops. Shake well, and apply to affected areas of skin.

Baths

If a child is calm, he or she will sleep better – and scratch less.

All the following bath methods will help induce calm and therefore sleep.

Oat bath

Put a handful of oatmeal or raw oats into a piece of material (such as muslin), and close securely. Drop the following essential oils on to the material:

chamomile german –
4 drops
lavender – 4 drops.

Attach the bundle to the tap, or hold it there, so the water gently runs through it before reaching the bath.

Salt bath

When the water has been run, add 1 tablespoon of sea salt to the bath, plus:

lavender – 1 drop
tea tree – 1 drop.

Soothing bath

Into 100g baking soda, add:

lavender – 2 drops
chamomile german –
1 drop.

Mix well with a spoon, before adding to the bath water.

Essential oils that help

lavender
chamomile german
chamomile roman

Anti-itching lotion

This lotion can be dabbed on to chickenpox spots after baths, or whenever needed.

Dab on the spots, allow to dry, then repeat.

Be careful to keep the lotion away from the eyes. Mix together:

60 ml (2 ounces) lavender hydrolat/water
60 ml (2 ounces) chamomile hydrolat/water
lavender (angustifolia) – 4 drops
chamomile german – 4 drops
eucalyptus radiata – 2 drops
ravensara – 2 drops.

Shake the ingredients together in a bottle; the essential oils will still float on the surface. Continue to shake vigorously, then pour through an unbleached coffee filter-paper into a measuring jug, then rebottle.

Other care

Calamine lotion is the traditionally used soothing preparation for this condition – spread it over the affected area and leave for a few hours, or overnight. The British Medical Association recommends soothing baths – essential oils can be added to vegetable oil, then put into bath water. Swish oil around well before the child gets in the bath.

If blisters are in the throat, have the child gargle with salt water to which a small amount of vinegar and honey has been added.

When to get help

It is wise to get a doctor's diagnosis as soon as possible. Call the doctor again if the child has any swelling or develops a cough or sore throat.

PREVENTION

 If a child has not yet had chickenpox, it's better not to carry out any preventative measures and
instead to allow the child to catch it. It's far better to have chickenpox in childhood than to catch
it for the first time as an adult – shingles can develop instead, a more serious and recurring
problem.

Circumcision

Circumcision is not a condition but a procedure. In boys, it's the surgical removal of the foreskin,
and is carried out under local anaesthetic (in Western countries, at least). The inner and outer
layers of the foreskin are removed, there are a few stitches, then a dressing is applied.
Circumcision may be carried out for medical reasons – perhaps the foreskin is too tight or there
are hygiene factors. More usually, it is a semi-religious ritual of both the Jewish and Muslim
traditions, sometimes performed by a rabbi or religious leader. In some groups it is performed
shortly after birth, while in others it occurs either before or at puberty – when he is often given
fabulous clothes to wear and receives gifts of money from relatives and friends.

Circumcision in girls is entirely different. In some countries, girls between 8 and 12 years of age
are cut around the genital area. Often with no anaesthetic or medical assistance, a traditional
healer or local woman practising female circumcision will remove some or all of the clitoris, also
possibly the labia minora and majora, and may even narrow the entrance to the vagina with
stitches.

Female circumcision has no religious basis (nor basis in religious writings). It's the women of the
community, including the mothers and grandmothers, who insist on continuing the practice.
They believe that girls will not be able to find a husband if they can't prove, by circumcision, that
their sexuality is under control and therefore their fidelity assured.

In 1980, it was estimated that 84 million women, in 30 African countries, had had circumcision
carried out on them. Some African mothers bring their daughters to the West to avoid them
having to endure the procedure. Although female circumcision is illegal in Western countries,
the tradition is still so strong that some doctors of the same culture, practising in the West,

clandestinely perform the procedure, when there is no valid medical reason for it. Complications can arise from these less professionally carried out cases.

Complications of the procedure

 infection

 redness; pain; swelling; pus

Method

Boys: infection prevention

First, prepare the antiseptic wash or spray for the area.

In 1 pint warm water, add 20 drops of lavender essential oil. Bottle, and shake very well. Now pour through a paper coffee-filter and rebottle.

Use before circumcision – as a rinse after washing, or in a spray, over the genital area.

Use after circumcision to also assist in healing, once the dressing has been removed.

Sitz baths (bowls in which you sit!)

For boys and girls

In a large plastic bowl full of warm water, add:

1 teaspoon salt
lavender – 7 drops.

Swish the water around well. Your child should sit in this sitz bath for 10 minutes or so.

Compresses

For boys and girls.

Use the compress method, made with:

lavender hydrolat
chamomile hydrolat.

Use one single hydrolat, or combine them.

Use a soft, muslin-type of material, folded over a few times. Soak it in the hydrolat, squeeze out well and then apply to the genitals.

Calming back rub

For girls

Make a calming body rub by mixing the following:

30 ml (1 ounce) vegetable oil
geranium – 5 drops
rose otto – 5 drops.

Use a small amount each time, to rub over your child's back. Do not use over the genital area.

Shock

For girls

See also *Shock* (page 239).

Essential oils that help

lavender
geranium
chamomile
rose otto

Other care

Use whatever traditional healing medicine is given in the circumstances, providing you know that it is effective.

When to get help

In both boys and girls, get immediate medical help if there is any sign of infection.

If, because of cultural pressure, circumcision has been carried out on your daughter, recently or in the past, legally or illegally, please seek professional medical care as soon as possible.

Cold sores ('fever blisters')

Cold sores are caused by the virus herpes simplex 1. They're caught by kissing someone who is infected, by sharing cups and utensils or some other contact. There may not be an outbreak of blisters with the initial infection, and the child may just have flu-like symptoms. Once caught, however, the cold sore virus will be with the child for their lifetime. According to American research, most affected people had their initial infection when they were between the ages of six months and 5 years.

The virus lives permanently on the nerve ending where initial contact was made. It may be dormant for the whole of the child's life, or there may be just one outbreak of blisters, or it could turn into a recurring problem. Certain conditions bring the virus out into the open. An outbreak of blisters is more likely to occur if the child is feeling nervous, if they are unwell, run-down, malnourished, if the weather is hot, or if they have another viral infection, such as flu, chickenpox, measles and the common cold – hence the term 'cold sores'.

Signs and symptoms

 small blisters that come up around the mouth, near the lips, or inside the mouth, on gums, throat, nostrils or elsewhere on the face

 blisters that eventually rupture, and crust over

 blisters that last 7–12 days

Cold sore mix

This is a mix of neat essential oil. It can be used on children over 2 years of age.

It can be applied to the area when the warning tingle is felt – before the cold sore erupts, or once it has already appeared. If the sore is open, this will sting, so warn your child before you put it on.

Use a fresh cotton-wool bud each time it touches the skin.

You will only use a small amount of the following each time:

chamomile german – 2 drops
geranium – 5 drops
tea tree – 5 drops.

Method

If you have a child with cold sores, there are two main things to remember. Cold sores come up at the same place, and before the blister appears there is a characteristic tingling in the area. If your child can learn to identify this advance signal, treatment can be given right away, which may even prevent the cold sore erupting. Also, the cold sores are very contagious – especially the fluid in the blister.

When a child has a cold sore, it's very important that the sore is not touched, because the infection could then be spread to other parts of the body that are touched afterwards. Your child should only use their own facecloth and towel, and should also avoid kissing.

Essential oils that help

lemon balm
lavender
tea tree
lemon
geranium
manuka
thyme linalol
chamomile german
melissa

Other care

Some people use surgical spirit to help to dry up the cold sores, although it does sting.
I personally wouldn't recommend this on any broken skin, but if you prefer this method, before using you could add a drop of lavender and 1 drop of tea tree to 1 drop of surgical spirit. If you use Vaseline or another type of mineral oil as a barrier method, you could add 8 drops each of manuka, thyme linalol and chamomile german to a 30g (1 ounce) tub of Vaseline, then mix well.

When to get help

Always consult your doctor to get a definite diagnosis. You should get further medical help if the eyes seem to be affected, as is the case sometimes; if there is a fever; or if the sores become infected with pus and are very red and painful. You should also tell your doctor if your child suffers from repeated cold sore eruptions.

Special note

Encephalitis can be caused by the herpes simplex 1 virus. If your child contracts encephalitis, tell your doctor that your child suffers from cold sores.

PREVENTION

If you or your child has a cold sore:

 Don't share facecloths, sponges, towels, cups, glasses or eating utensils.

 Try to stop your child touching the cold sore.

 Change pillows or bedlinen every day, to prevent cross-infection.

 If hot weather makes the cold sore erupt, use double the amount of sun screen , particularly on the lips.

Colds (the common cold)

Colds are perhaps the most common ailment of both children and adults. They are an infection by various types of viruses, all contagious. A child of any age can catch a cold but it's especially distressing for babies, who experience difficulty in drinking from a bottle or breast when they have a stuffed-up nose.

Antibiotics cannot treat colds. They are best avoided at this time because the child's tolerance of them may build up, so when antibiotics are *really* needed, a higher dose will be necessary.

Signs and symptoms

   runny nose, stuffed nose

   congestion – often on the chest

   cough

   fever

Method

Foot massage for chills

If the child has a chill that makes him or her feel cold and shivery, massage both feet with the following mix before bedtime:	1 teaspoon vegetable oil ginger – 1 drop ormenis flower (chamomile maroc) – 1 drop.	Ensure the child has enough bedclothes.

The colds mix

This blend of essential oils can be used in a variety of methods. Mix the oils in these proportions and bottle for when needed:

eucalyptus radiata – 10 drops
ravensara – 10 drops
tea tree – 5 drops
lavender – 3 drops
thyme linalol – 1 drop.

Baths
Dilute the colds mix (see above) in vegetable oil before adding it to a bath. Use the following amounts of colds mix, according to the age of the child, in 1 teaspoon vegetable oil:

2–18 months	1 drop
19 months–3 years	2 drops
4–6 years	3 drops
7–11 years	4 drops
12 years and over	5 drops.

For babies under 2 months, put 1 drop of the colds mix in 2 teaspoons vegetable oil, blend well, and use only ¹/₂ teaspoon per bath.

Tissue
Put 2 drops of the colds mix on a tissue. The child can sniff from this to help relieve the symptoms.

Inhalation
This method should only be used by children who are old enough to understand the danger of hot water. See Chapter 3 for directions.

Use 3 drops of the colds mix per inhalation.

Steam method
This method is effective with babies. Again, see Chapter 3 for directions. Place the bowl of steaming water near or under the baby's cot. Add 3 drops of the colds mix.

Baby massage
Only use a very tiny amount of the following mix each time.

Massage into the upper chest and back at each nappy change:

2 teaspoons vegetable oil
colds mix - 1 drop.

Sinus massage

This can only be used on children over 3 years of age.

Smooth a tiny amount of the following mix over the nose, sinus area of the upper cheek and above the eyebrows. Use very little at a time, being careful the oil does not go near the eyes, and wipe any excess off with a tissue. This can be done after the child has fallen asleep. Use only a very small amount of this mix each application.

1 tablespoon vegetable oil
lemon – 2 drops
niaouli – 1 drop
colds mix (see above) – 5 drops.

Essential oils that help

tea tree
eucalyptus radiata
thyme linalol
manuka
ravensara
niaouli

Other care

Keep your child warm, snug and calm. Fresh air is a far better atmosphere for the child than bacteria-laden warm air, so open the windows when your child leaves a room, to keep the home healthily ventilated. Use a mix of anti-bacterial essential oils in a diffuser (see the list on page 11). Make sure your child drinks plenty of fluids.

When to get help

Get medical advice if your child has a temperature over 38.9° C (102° F) with or without a fever, if they complain of earache and neck pain, or if their difficult breathing does not seem to improve.

PREVENTION

 Keep babies away from people who have colds or are sneezing.

 Colds very often pass from person to person within the home. Spray rooms frequently with anti-viral essential oils and ask anyone at home with a cold to try to keep away from the children until the cold has passed.

 If colds are going around your child's school, send him or her in with a tissue on which you have put 2 drops of the colds mix. The child can sniff from this during the day. Tell other parents/carers what you are doing, as they might want to join you in this preventative measure.

Colic

Infantile colic is quite common, and in some cases can go on for many months. It's very painful for the baby, and highly distressing for the parents. Babies can be affected whether they're fed from the breast or the bottle. Colic is usually eased when trapped gas is eventually passed, or a bowel movement is made.

Why some babies should get colic, and others not, is still something of a mystery. There are many theories including: *what* the mother eats, if she's breastfeeding; *how* the baby eats; and what measures are taken to 'wind' the baby after he or she has eaten. All may be contributing to the condition. However, even when all these things are done perfectly, babies can and do still get colic, and cry . . . and cry . . . and cry!

Colic, of course, is not the only reason babies cry – check first that your baby is not hungry or in need of a nappy change. However, although there seems to be an expectation that 'all babies cry', there may be a serious underlying problem that needs medical attention.

Signs and symptoms

 intense crying, which can go on for hours, usually in the late afternoon or early evening

 baby's abdomen feels hard to the touch

 flushed face; lips might become pale

 baby may draw legs up to stomach and/or clench fists

Method

If winding doesn't work, mothers often intuitively massage over the baby's abdomen to help release the trapped gas. This is best done gently in small circular movements, 5–10 minutes after feeding or winding. It can be done while the baby is clothed.

Essential oils can be used in a massage oil for the baby. Lay your baby down on your knees and remove any restrictive clothing, including the nappy. Using no more than ¼ teaspoon of the mix at a time, gently massage the abdomen in small, clockwise, circular movements, then turn the baby over and massage the centre of the back, again in small, clockwise circles. Baby may be uncomfortable with the massage on the abdomen, but do persist. When massaging the back, you could place your baby on a towel that's been warmed on a radiator, but make sure it's not hot. If the legs are drawn up, you could try massaging the legs and the feet.

Massage oil

First, mix the essential oils using these proportions:

coriander – 5 drops
cardamom – 3 drops
dill – 2 drops.

Bottle the essential oils for future use. When required, mix 1 drop only in $1/2$ teaspoon almond oil – use half this amount per application.

Baths

To help relax the spasm, add $1/4$ teaspoon of the following mix to a warm bath:

1 teaspoon almond oil
lavender – 1 drop
cardamom – 1 drop.

Put the $1/4$ teaspoon mix in the bath; it will float on the surface. Scoop it into your hand and rub over baby's tummy while in the bath. Make sure none splashes into baby's eyes.

Dill herb water

Add 1 teaspoon of the following mixture to 120 ml (4 ounces) slightly warm, boiled water in a bottle, for baby to drink.

Put the following in a small bowl:

1 handful fresh dill herb
1 handful fresh mint herb
$1/4$ teaspoon fennel seeds.

Pour $1/2$ pint boiling water over these, then add 1 teaspoon of honey, mix a little, cover with a plate and leave to cool. Strain, then bottle.
See above – use only 1 teaspoon of the mixture in 120 ml (4 ounces) water.

Essential oils that help

cardamon
dill
coriander

When to get help

On the whole, colic eases after a baby reaches around 4 months old. If it doesn't, help should be sought. A baby with unusual bowel movements could have intestinal problems, so a doctor should be consulted. If baby vomits up his or her food on a regular basis, again you should get some help. And, if the vomiting is projectile (that is, it comes out of the mouth with force and travels some distance), this can indicate a serious problem and medical attention should be sought immediately.

PREVENTION

  If breastfeeding, the mother could try reducing her intake of caffeine and/or fizzy drinks, dairy products, onions, garlic, cabbage and spicy foods.

  After feeding and winding, put 1 drop of dill essential oil on a tissue and tuck it under the baby's mattress – at the end opposite to baby's head.

Computer-related problems

Computers have not been around long enough for physiologists and psychologists to evaluate fully the effect they have on our children as they enter adulthood and, eventually, their senior years. Many children today are becoming obsessed with the computer, and spend far too long on it. Some parents tell me their children won't eat unless food is taken to them while they sit at the computer, chatting on email or playing games. Some children are spending all their free time at the computer, as well as using them at school. This can lead to various problems, especially if the child is accessing information their parents would disapprove of.

Parents are perhaps most worried about the type of information available on the internet – especially of a sexual or violent nature. But the PC can be the source of other, more physical concerns, including radiation, in terms of electrical and magnetic emissions – including ELF (extremely low emissions) and VLF (magnetic fields, electrical fields, static electricity fields). Studies have shown that these magnetic fields do have biological effects, particularly on the growth of various cells and tissue, hormones, and brain chemicals and functioning.

Working at a PC for long periods also causes obvious physical problems, such as repetitive strain from working on the keyboard with the fingers and hands, visual disturbance caused by the glare of the VDU screen, tinnitus and other hearing problems caused by the continual low buzz of the hard disk drive, and asthma exacerbated by an increased number of dust particles in the dry atmosphere.

The two following lists outline the psychological and physical problems that may affect children who spend too long on the computer.

Signs and symptoms

Emotional

 non-communication

 irritability

 abusiveness

 distancing themselves from family

 'nobody understands me' syndrome

 sadness

 having no feelings

 emotional outbursts for no apparent reason

 hopelessness

 insomnia

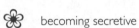

❀ becoming secretive

❀ getting up to chat online when the family have gone to bed

Stress

❀ irritability

❀ grinding teeth

❀ muscle tension

❀ fatigue – but unable to sleep

❀ changes in appetite

❀ aggression

❀ shallow breathing

Method

> ### Room diffuser or spray
>
> Use essential oils in the room methods when your child is at the computer. If using the spray method, make sure none of the water droplets fall on to the computer or keyboard. The best oils to use at this time are those extracted from leaves and trees and which oxygenate the atmosphere, such as:
>
> petitgrain, cypress, pine and fir.
>
> Also consider using the following:
>
> eucalyptus – to help with the radiation and assist in breathing
> lavender – to help insomnia
> lemon – to help focus and concentration while completing school projects and homework.

Other care

Limit the length of time younger children spend on the computer, and make sure your child's computer has a glare-control screen. Ensure no reflected light is appearing on the screen, and reorganize room lighting so your child's eyes are not being strained. Your child should sit on a well-designed ergonomic chair, with a backrest, and work with elbows on the desk, supporting the wrists. Most emissions come out of the back of the computer, so make sure it backs on to an external wall, and not a seating or sleeping area. Radiation increases in dry, hot places, so make sure the air is humid, and put plants in the room such as the peace lily or spider plant – both easily available, even in supermarkets.

Increase your child's intake of vitamins C and E, as ELF (extremely low frequency) emissions are thought to increase the incidence of free radicals (molecules thought to be responsible for many diseases and disorders) in the body. Give your child lots to drink while he or she is working on the computer, making sure no cups or cans are put on the computer desk, where they can be knocked on to the keyboard.

PREVENTION

 There was a time when we could see who our child was talking to, and take steps to prevent that association if we disapproved. With the advent of internet and emails, those days have gone. Even the children themselves don't know who they're 'talking' to, and paedophiles may be masquerading as children in internet 'chatrooms'. In truth, we don't know who is at the end of the line, or what thoughts they are putting into our child's head. Moreover, the internet is full of all kinds of information – some educational, and some very dangerous. Have we any idea what our child is learning through it? Spend time with your child on the computer, asking what he or she has found on the internet. If you can talk about it together, it may prevent a 'them and us' situation – 'they' the parents don't know what's going on, while 'we' kids do.

We must also ask ourselves as parents if we encourage our children to use the computer because we feel secure knowing where they are – rather than on the street, getting into gangs, meeting the wrong people and drinking or taking drugs, perhaps. Are we encouraging our children to make friends on the computer instead of encouraging them to interact with real-life human beings?

Constipation

Although constipation is usually considered to be the absence of stools for a time, it's more accurately defined as stools with a hard (pebble-like) texture. It can be caused by a change in dietary habits, stress or earlier toilet training. Babies often have constipation when eating solids for the first time. If the child has a fever, the stools may be harder than normal, because the body absorbs fluid from wherever it can in order to compensate for the lack of water in the body.

Signs and symptoms

 dry, hard stools – pebble-like

 stools difficult to pass

Method

Tummy rub

First, feel around your child's lower abdomen to see if there is any tenderness in the area. If there is, see your doctor straight away. If all is well, prepare the following mix:

1 teaspoon vegetable oil
mandarin – 2 drops
lemon – 2 drops
petitgrain – 1 drop.

Use a small amount each time. Massage the whole of your child's abdomen in gentle movements, working around the umbilicus (tummy button) in a clockwise direction.

Essential oils that help

mandarin
petitgrain
lemon
grapefruit

Other care

Give your child plenty of plain water to drink – sweetened with a little honey, if necessary. Let your child's body pass the stools in its own time; don't say it is necessary to go to the toilet at a certain regular time of day. Teach your child to take time on the toilet or potty. To prevent boredom, read a story, perhaps get him or her to read to you, or listen to music together – do anything to encourage your child to stay put, particularly if he or she is very active.

When to get help

Check your child's lower abdomen to see if there is any tenderness in the area. If there is, see your doctor straight away. Also get medical help if there's any blood in the stools, or stomach pains, or if the constipation lasts for longer than five days.

PREVENTION

 Give your child plenty of water to drink.

 Get your child to eat lots of fibre – prunes, fruit, cereal, bran, bananas, sweetcorn and wholemeal bread, for example.

Cough

See also Asthma; Bronchitis; Croup; Tonsillitis; Whooping cough.

Coughing is not a condition as such – it's a symptom of some other problem within the body. The coughing reflex is the body trying to clear irritating material from the throat or airways, and is proof that the body's defence system is working as it should. We all cough sometimes, but when it is excessive we know something is wrong.

Signs and symptoms

 sound, depth and source of the cough can indicate where the body's defence system is working – and where the cause of the trouble is located

 cough may come from the chest or the throat

 cough sounds like gurgling as mucus is removed from the airways

Method

Cough mix

This cough mix can be used in several ways. Mix the following oils, using these proportions, and bottle:

ravensara – 10 drops
niaouli – 5 drops
eucalyptus radiata – 10 drops.

Chest and back rub
Rub over the chest and back. Dilute the chest mix of essential oils above in 1 tablespoon vegetable oil, using the following amounts, depending on the age of the child. Only use a small amount of your diluted oil each time you apply.

under 2 years	4 drops
3–7 years	6 drops
8–11 years	8 drops.

This can be used throughout the day, but just before bed is the most effective time.

The rub may help the body loosen any mucus, so the coughing may temporarily get worse as the body rids itself of the mucus, as part of the healing process.

Steam bowl

To help your child breathe easily during the night, put 8 drops of the cough mix of essential oils into a bowl of steaming-hot water. Leave in the child's room as he or she goes to sleep. Place out of reach, and keep pets away until the water has cooled down a little.

Tissue, pillow or pyjamas
To help the child breathe easily during the night, put one drop of the cough mix of essential oils on:

 a tissue and tuck under the pillow; or
 on the pillow, away from the eye area; or
 on the chest area of the pyjamas.

Essential oils that help

eucalyptus radiata
niaouli
ravensara
thyme linalol
chamomile german

Essential oils that help aid sleep

lavender
neroli
ormenis flower (chamomile maroc)

Other care

Keep your child warm, and give plenty to drink. He or she should avoid doing highly active games or sports, and stay away from areas where people are smoking. Moist air can be very helpful – use a humidifier or, if you don't have one, put a small bowl of steaming-hot water in the child's room – out of reach of children and pets – or put a wet towel or other cloth over a hot radiator.

When to get help

All children under a year old who have a cough should be examined by a doctor. If the child is more than a year, get medical advice if the coughing lasts for longer than 24 hours, or if there is a temperature or fever, or if the child has difficulty in breathing in or out. If a cough lasts over one week, visit your doctor.

Cradle cap (Seborrhoea dermatitis)

Cradle cap is a skin irritation that affects babies. It's caused by overactivity of the sebacceous glands and dead skin, which creates a build-up of a greasy crust on the scalp. It gets worse with perspiration, so keep the head dry, cool and open to the air whenever possible.

Do not try to remove the crust with your fingers, or rub the scalp vigorously. Instead, brush the hair with a very soft baby's brush. Whatever method you use to treat the condition, it could take up to two weeks to clear completely. Only give treatment while the condition exists.

Method

Aromatherapy

Only use a small amount each time. Gently smooth over the scalp to help loosen scales. Mix together:

15 ml (^{1}/2 ounce) avocado oil
15 ml (^{1}/2 ounce) jojoba oil
tea tree –1 drop
orange oil –1 drop
lemon oil –1 drop.

Leave for a few minutes, then shampoo off with a mild shampoo. Be careful not to get the oil or shampoo in baby's eye or face.

Tea wash

Add 1 teaspoon of the following 'tea' to the final rinse water when washing baby's hair:

^{1}/2 pint water
juice of half a lemon
1 handful fresh rosemary
1 handful fresh thyme.

Put the herbs in a bowl with the lemon juice. Boil the water and pour over the herbs. Leave until cold, then bottle.

Plain oil

Try to use cold-pressed organic oils such as almond or sunflower oil. Only use a small amount each time, gently smoothing the oil over the scalp to help loosen scales.

Signs and symptoms

  can occur on the head, in the eyebrows and even behind the ears

  dry, scaly patches becoming flaky

  soft, crusty, thick yellow scales; can become hard and thick

Essential oils that help

tea tree
geranium
lemon
orange

When to get help

A scaly scalp can be caused by eczema, psoriasis or ringworm. If you suspect any of these, consult your doctor. Also, consult your doctor if the scales last longer than two or three weeks, if they become reddened, or if there are scaly patches in places other than the head, eyebrows or behind the ears.

Croup

See also Colds (the common cold); Cough; Laryngitis.

The main symptom of croup is a strange cough that sounds rather like a seal barking – a kind of croaking. The most likely cause is an infection of the airways, but a croaking sound can also be made if the child has swallowed an object that has got stuck in the throat.

The infection is usually caused by a virus, which makes the upper part of the airways swollen. When the air passes through the airways, it causes the strange sound and cough. Croup can follow an infection like bronchitis. It mostly affects children between 6 months and 3 years old.

Signs and symptoms

 often starts during the night, when it can seem worse

 difficulty in breathing; chest seems to be deflating more than usual

 high-pitched wheezing noise (stridor) when the child inhales

 (often) sore throat, hoarse voice; fever

 possible gagging/vomiting

 irritability and tiredness

Method

Steamy room

The only practical way to get a room full of steam is to run a very hot bath in the bathroom, with the door tightly shut. Put a chair in the room, where you can sit with your child on your knee. This is a good time to read a book to him or her – do not leave your child alone. Add the following essential oils to the hot bath water:

niaouli – 10 drops
eucalyptus radiata – 10 drops.

This bath is not intended to bathe in: the aim is to create an essential oil steamy atmosphere for your child to inhale.

Croup mix

First, mix these essential oils together:

niaouli – 15 drops
ravensara – 15 drops
thyme linalol – 10 drops
palmarosa – 10 drops.

The mix can be used in the two methods below.

Chest and back massage

Dilute 3 drops of the croup mix of essential oils in 1 tablespoon vegetable oil. Only use a small amount of this each time – to massage over the chest and back.

Pillow or pyjamas

Put 1 drop of the croup mix of essential oils:

❋   **on the pillow, away from the eye area; or**

❋   **on the chest area of the pyjamas.**

Essential oils that help

eucalyptus radiata
niaouli
ravensara
thyme linalol
chamomile german
palmarosa

Essential oils that help aid sleep
lavender
neroli
marjoram
chamomile maroc

Other care

Cool, moist evening air appears to help during attacks, but if the child is going out, make sure he or she is well wrapped up and warm. At night, add more pillows so your child is propped up in bed. Try to stay calm during a coughing attack – it's bad enough for the child and it doesn't help if he or she sees that you are completely panicky!

When to get help

If you think your child's cough is a result of having swallowed something, call emergency services straight away.

Consult your doctor if your child has a temperature, if his or her face has a greyish colour, or he or she cannot breathe, refuses to drink liquids, or if the cough continues more than three days. It may be necessary for your child to have oxygen.

PREVENTION

 Keep your child off school if he or she has bronchitis or shows sign of a respiratory infection. Make every effort to deal with the infection during this time.

Cuts and grazes – minor

Children are forever getting themselves into minor accidents as they leap about the place – and cuts and grazes are often the result. Some cuts bleed quite a lot, and until they stop you don't really know the extent of the damage. A deep cut will need to be sutured – stitched up by a professional – and ideally this should be carried out within eight hours. Most usually, though, children suffer minor cuts and grazes, which can be treated at home.

If there's a lot of bleeding, apply pressure to the area with a clean, absorbent piece of material to help stop the flow. If the cut is on a limb, hold the injured part up for a while, to lessen blood flow to the area.

Signs and symptoms

 cuts – there's a break in the skin, usually with some bleeding

 cuts – a puncture of the skin caused by the removal of a splinter or other object

 grazes – the top layer of skin has been removed by scraping on a hard surface (this may ooze a fluid, or bleed slightly in spots)

Method

Cuts and grazes mix

You can pretty much guarantee that if there's a child in the home you'll need some cuts and grazes mix. Bottle these simple ingredients up for when the need arises:

lavender – 50 drops
tea tree – 50 drops.

Washing

With all cuts and grazes, it's extremely important to remove all traces of dirt or grit, and the only way this can be done is by washing the area thoroughly. The child may not like it, but it has to be done. Use warm water, and if there's dirt inside the cut, flush it out using any super-clean utensil that suits the job.

Add 10 drops of the cuts and grazes mix to the water you use to wash the area. It is antiseptic, and will calm your child down.

Gauze dressing

Put 3 drops of the cuts and grazes mix on a gauze dressing and let it dry. Alternatively, use lavender on its own. Place that dressing directly over the cut or graze, then bandage it up.

Expose the cut or graze to the air as much as possible, and apply the gauze dressing twice a day.

Plaster dressing

Put 1 drop of the cuts and grazes mix (or 1 drop of lavender) on to the dressing part of the plaster, which will cover the wounded area. Let it dry before applying.

Don't put the essential oils directly on the cut itself – this will sting and it is unnecessary.

Aftercare

Change the dressing often, and leave the wound exposed to the air as much as possible. If the grazed area is very large, use the gauze dressing method.

To help with the healing process and keep infection at bay, smear 1 drop of the cuts and grazes mix (or lavender) in a circle surrounding the cut or graze. Apply it on unbroken skin around the area, not directly on the cut or graze.

If there is swelling, wrap a few ice cubes in a towel and hold it against the affected area.

Essential oils that help

lavender
pine
tea tree
lemon
manuka
eucalyptus radiata
niaouli

When to get help

Go for medical help straightaway if the wound seems to be more than half an inch deep into the tissue; or if the cut is jagged and cannot be cleaned properly; or if the bleeding does not stop after 10 minutes of applying pressure with a clean cloth or dressing.

Get medical help if the wound does not heal, or if an infection develops and there is pus, swelling or more tenderness and redness in the area than before, and possibly a fever.

If you see any red lines extending outwards from the cut or graze, do not hesitate, and go immediately to your doctor.

PREVENTION

 There's not much you can do to prevent children having cuts and grazes – that's kids for you! What you can do is help prevent your child getting tetanus, by making sure he or she has regular injections. Check with your doctor that your child's tetanus immunization is up-to-date.

Dandruff

See also Cradle cap (Seborrhoea dermatitis).

Children get dandruff for different reasons. It may just be a build-up of cells on the scalp, or it could be a sign of eczema, psoriasis or a fungal infection. Head lice are a parasitic infestation of the scalp, and the empty eggshells left by the small creatures can look very much like dandruff. Children of all ages get dandruff, which can sometimes also affect the eyebrows.

Signs and symptoms

 white flakes of dead skin on the scalp and hair, which fall on to the shoulders

 dead skin attached to the scalp, which if not removed can build up into crusty areas

Method

Sometimes, when medication and medicated dandruff shampoos are stopped, the symptoms return and even increase, so the product must be bought again to keep the symptoms at bay.

This is no long-term solution. As an alternative, try the following, natural three-part dandruff plan. It needs to be carried out once a week, with no other washes in between – removing the build-up of dandruff with constant washing only seems to encourage the shedding of more skin cells. Instead, leave it alone and see if the scalp can balance itself out.

The three-part dandruff plan

The oil

Mix the following to make an oil to use at night:

30 ml (1 ounce) jojoba oil
8 ml (¼ ounce) rosehip oil
red carrot oil – 15 drops.

Use only a small amount, but make sure it covers all the scalp. Rub it in well.

This mix may stain your bedlinen, so use an old pillowcase. In the morning, use the shampoo.

The shampoo

Shampoo the oil off in the morning. Use the gentlest, most natural shampoo you can find – there are products for babies, children or non-perfumed brands for sensitive skin. Ideally, use a shampoo that uses coconut derivatives, or the foaming agent from soap wort, rather than other detergents. Essential oils can be mixed directly in with the shampoo. The following amounts are for 4 fluid ounces of shampoo:

tea tree – 10 drops
manuka – 10 drops
myrtle – 5 drops.

Then rinse.

The final rinse

After shampooing, rinse the hair thoroughly. Then apply this final rinse, which you leave in the hair. The following amount would be enough for at least eight final rinses:

250 ml (8 ounces) water
lemon – 26 drops
tea tree – 5 drops.

Shake well, then pour through an unbleached paper coffee-filter, and bottle for future use.

Essential oils that help

myrtle

tea tree

manuka

lemon

cypress

red carrot seed

Other oils that help

jojoba

borage

almond

rosehip seed

When to get help

Get medical advice if the child has eczema or psoriasis anywhere on the body, or if there is a fungal skin infection, or if you suspect head lice.

Dehydration

The body is made up of 80 per cent water, which helps to move vital nutrients around the body. When the body is starved of water, we quickly deteriorate, so if a child vomits, has diarrhoea or a fever, precious fluids are being lost – and dehydration can result.

The most obvious reason a child becomes dehydrated is because he or she has not been drinking enough. Pure water is by far the best liquid for children, and they do like it, if offered. Pure fruit juice is sugar-laden, but it can be diluted down with water. Other drinks contain artificial sweeteners, caffeine, and chemicals for colour, preservative and flavour – which aren't exactly known for doing the body any good.

Dehydration is serious. Any child with vomiting and diarrhoea should be given immediate medical help – both to help rid the body of whatever infection is causing the symptoms, and to get the right levels of fluid back into the body.

Signs and symptoms

   dry lips and mouth

   vomiting or diarrhoea that lasts more than five hours

   drowsiness; sleepiness

   (sometimes) dark and smelly urine – when it becomes clearer, that's a good sign

Method

If your child gets dehydrated, for whatever reason, give him or her frequent sips of water – even if it does pass straight through the body. If no water is available, give whatever fluid you have.

If you are taking your child camping or hiking, or for some other reason away from a city with medical facilities, make sure you purchase a rehydration mixture or carry the crucial ingredients of a dehydration fluid (see right), just in case the child gets sick while away. Don't even think about cutting out the sugar or glucose – that's needed to aid absorption of the salt.

Dehydration drink

Sip one glass at a time.

1 pint water
$^1/_2$ teaspoon salt
4 teaspoons glucose powder (or 6 teaspoons sugar)

Stir until dissolved. Add a little fruit juice if the child refuses to drink the dehydration mix on its own.

Other care

Make your child sip drinks – drinking too quickly is not good because your child's stomach may reject the liquid. Little and often is the rule for dehydration. Don't allow your child to overheat: keep him or her between cool and warm.

When to get help

As soon as you can.

Diarrhoea

See also Dehydration.

Diarrhoea is the name given to runny, loose stools. It could be caused by many things, including bacterial and viral stomach infections, stress or an allergic reaction to a food or medication. Diarrhoea is a possible symptom of many conditions, including colds, flu, ear infection and sore throats. If it continues for a long time, your child may become dehydrated.

Young babies, particularly if breastfed, may have soft stools – but this is normal. If your child has no symptoms other than a bout of diarrhoea, don't worry, as it will probably pass. If your child is continually passing loose stools (even after a drink of water), seek help, as this is not normal.

Signs and symptoms

 variously coloured runny stools

 fluid being passed anally

Method

Tummy rubs

Use a small amount, to rub over the whole of your child's abdominal area.

Choose from the appropriate mix.

Viral infection
Dilute the following essential oils in 1 tablespoon vegetable oil:

thyme linalol – 3 drops
lavender – 2 drops
tea tree – 1 drop.

Use a small amount each time.

Food poisoning
Dilute the following essential oils in 1 tablespoon vegetable oil:

chamomile german – 2 drops
peppermint – 3 drops
eucalyptus radiata – 1 drop.

Use a small amount each time.

Stress
Dilute the following essential oils in 1 tablespoon vegetable oil:

chamomile roman – 1 drop
eucalyptus radiata – 2 drops
lavender – 3 drops.

Use a small amount each time.

Back rub for calm and sleep

The following mix will help your child to sleep if they are distressed:

1 teaspoon vegetable oil
lavender – 1 drop
petitgrain – 1 drop.

Use half this amount if your child is under 3 years of age.

Apply on your child's back, and gently rub in.

Essential oils that help, if it's caused by

Viral infection	Food poisoning	Stress
tea tree	thyme linalol	lavender
lemon	tea tree	geranium
lavender	eucalyptus radiata	lemon
eucalyptus radiata	chamomile german	chamomile roman
thyme linalol	peppermint	
lavender		

Other care

Let the diarrhoea take its course – it may be the body getting rid of a virus or bacteria. To help rehydrate your child's body, give small sips of an electrolyte solution (available from chemists), and supply plenty of water to drink during the day.

When to get help

See your doctor as soon as possible if there is blood in the stools, stomach pain, vomiting, temperature or fever. Also get help if the diarrhoea lasts longer than 10 hours.

PREVENTION

 Food poisoning and diarrhoea are sometimes caused by poor hygiene. Teach the whole family to wash their hands before touching or preparing foods.

Earache and ear infection

These are both very common in childhood, and can be extremely painful. They can affect children of all ages, and are as common as colds in those under 5 years of age. Considering the events leading up to the pain is important when trying to identify the cause, because this will help decide what treatment is appropriate. An infection may lead to earache, but you need to ask yourself if was it caused by a cold, tonsillitis or mumps, or by having water in the ear, which then became infected. Other causes of earache are toothache and sinus problems – and that might be sinusitis or hayfever-related. Having a boil or spot in the area can cause earache, as can being out in the cold, wind or snow. So, try to narrow down the reason for the earache, and tell this to your doctor or treat accordingly.

If your child has recurring earaches for no apparent reason, it's likely they have an infection that is not responding to treatment. All earaches should be treated as a potential long-term problem because, if they're left untreated, hearing in later life might be impaired. If the pain is persistent, it could indicate a perforated eardrum, or an infection.

Signs and symptoms

 pain

 discharge or fluid coming out of the ear indicates an infection

 fever; colds and sniffles; irritability; balance problems

 in very young children – pulling or rubbing the ears, crying, distress

 in older children – dizziness

Method

Ear massage

Massage around the back of the affected ear – outside the ear, on the side of the head – with one of the following mixes:

Earache mix
Use only a small amount each time.

15 ml (¹/2 ounce) vegetable oil
lavender – 10 drops
chamomile german – 5 drops
palmarosa – 6 drops
cardamom – 3 drops.

Ear infection mix 1
Use only a small amount each time. If this is not effective, try the (stronger) mix number 2 (below).

15 ml (¹/2 ounce) vegetable oil
thyme linalol – 3 drops
lavender – 3 drops

Ear infection mix 2
First, mix up these essential oils:

thyme linalol – 5 drops
lavender – 3 drops

chamomile roman – 10 drops
palmarosa – 3 drops.

Use 3 drops of this mix, diluted in 1 teaspoon vegetable oil, but use only ¹/2 teaspoon.

Ear infection compress
A warm compress may help with the pain. Put 3 drops of thyme linalol and 3 drops of lavender on a warm compress, and hold against the ear.

Essential oils that help ear infection

niaouli
marjoram
juniper berry
tea tree
thyme linalol
lavender
chamomile roman

Other care

Warmth sometimes helps to soothe earache. Do this by holding a covered hot-water bottle against the ear, or by putting a heated-up, covered, wheat bag in the child's pillowcase. Wheat bags are herb or grain bags that can be heated in the microwave. They can be bought in health food shops and some department stores. Don't use these methods if boils or spots are present.

When to get help

The causes of earache have the potential to be harmful to the child's health, and it's important to get a proper diagnosis. Always get medical advice if there is any loss of hearing, discharge from the ear, high temperature, fever, loss of balance, if your child has a red and sore throat, spots and boils, or if the pain has continued for more than 24 hours.

Eczema (atopic dermatitis)

Eczema is an itchy skin condition that is often caused by an allergy to certain foods or environmental factors. It often starts to develop at the time solid foods are introduced into the diet, at around four or five months of age. If it occurs before then, the child may be allergic to powdered milk, or to breast milk – particularly if it contains allergy-producing elements. Most children with infantile eczema grow out of it by the age of 3, but for some unlucky children it can continue into adulthood.

Eczema is closely associated with asthma and hayfever, and the child may have these conditions as well. There is also a genetic factor – if either parent, or the grandparents, have these conditions, it may be expressed in the child as eczema.

If the eczema is allergy-based, the most likely sources of the trouble are wheat, dairy produce, eggs, pet hair, wool, water-softening agents and clothes-softening products. Eczema can also be triggered by stress and anxiety.

Signs and symptoms

   dry, flaky skin; cracking of the skin; scaly skin

   itching skin; redness

   red rash mainly affecting face, armpits, knees, elbows, hands, genital area

Note: fragrance can cause sensitivity; carry out a small skin test 24 hours before using essential oils.

Method

Soothing baths

Scratching makes the itch worse, and can cause infection. One of the best ways to reduce the irritation is to have soothing baths. There are several types to choose from:

Vegetable oil bath
Add 1 tablespoon plain vegetable oil to a bath. It will float on the surface, and moisten the child's skin when he or she comes out of the bath.

Don't use anything with wheatgerm in it, or any other oil produced from a grain.

Use one of the following:

almond oil
jojoba oil
grapeseed oil
sunflower seed oil.

Anxiety-relieving bath
To the vegetable oil used in the method to the left, add 2 or 3 drops of either lavender or geranium oil.

Oat-bag bath
To make your own oat bag, put a small number of organic oats on a square of muslin material.

Drop on to the oats:
$1/2$ teaspoon jojoba oil
lavender – 1 drop.

Tie the bag securely, and place in the bath.

Soothing lotions

Oil mix
Use a small amount of the following oil mix on the affected areas of skin, as needed. First, mix the following essential oils together:

lavender – 10 drops
chamomile german – 10 drops
palmarosa – 6 drops
bergamot – 2 drops.

Then, mix the following vegetable oils together:

60 ml (2 ounces) almond oil
8 ml ($^1/_4$ ounce) jojoba oil
15 ml ($^1/_2$ ounce) sunflower seed oil
8 ml ($^1/_4$ ounce) camellia oil
evening primrose oil – 6 drops.

Now combine the essential oil mix and the vegetable oil mix.

Calamine lotion mix
To each 120 ml (4 ounces) calamine lotion, add 2 drops of your chosen essential oil. See the list below.

Essential oils that help

chamomile german
elemi
yarrow
ho wood
lavender
palmarosa

Other care

Use calamine lotion, with or without essential oils. Avoid astringent lotions and mineral-based baby oils.

When to get help

As soon as the first sign of eczema appears, make a note of everything new your child has been exposed to, as he or she may be allergic to some element in its manufacture. Ask yourself whether new food or drinks have been consumed, or a new piece of clothing worn. Also, note whether you have used a new clothes detergent or household cleaner. If an allergy is involved, it could be caused by something very unobvious, like a new pillow, whether feather or foam. Think of everything new that you can, take it out of the child's environment and see if things improve.

Epilepsy – seizures

The seizures of epilepsy can affect children to varying degrees. Petit mal seizures are the less dramatic kind, with slight shaking and/or the child going into a trance-like state for a time; while grand mal seizures overtake the whole body, and the child may thrash about uncontrollably for several minutes.

Signs and symptoms

    uncontrolled body movements, over a period of minutes

    slight shaking; faraway look

Method

Brain-wave imaging systems have proved that essential oils do have an effect on seizures. At the Queen Elizabeth Hospital in Birmingham, Dr Tim Betts and his team have had great success in reducing patients' epilepsy seizures using the essential oils of jasmine, ylang ylang, chamomile and lavender. The other oils on the list below would work equally well.

Whether carried out professionally, or at home by parents and carers, aromatherapy treatment should be calming, and consistent – using repeatedly the same essential oil. Dr Betts' work has shown that, after a time and use of a particular essential oil or blend, patients who suffer from seizures may simply be able to sniff from a bottle of the same essential oil or blend used in treatment in order to prevent seizures from happening while they are out and about enjoying life.

Massage oil

Use the following volumes to make the massage oil:

30 ml (1 ounce) vegetable oil
essential oil – 5 drops.

Do not be tempted to use more essential oil than this. It's unnecessary, and it is better to use small amounts with this condition.

Only use a little of the oil at a time, to massage the child's back, just before sleep. Use upward-stroking movements, towards the neck. Do this twice a week to start with, gradually reducing the number of massages.

While massaging your child, play a tape of gentle music, or relaxing sounds such as woodland birdsong or a stream of water.

If the oils you have chosen are having a positive effect in reducing the incidence of seizures, give your child a tissue with a drop of that same essential oil. He or she can use it to sniff whenever they feel a seizure might be coming on, or when feeling anxious.

Essential oils that help

jasmine
petitgrain
neroli
chamomile roman
rose
geranium

Fever

Fever is the body's reaction to some other cause, and is a symptom, rather than an illness. There are many things it could be symptomatic of: in babies, it could be because a tooth is coming through. A fever might result from flu, a cold, cough, tonsillitis, chickenpox, measles, mumps, food poisoning, or earache – anything that's been caused by bacteria or a virus. It's the body trying to fight off an infection, a natural process that is, nonetheless, very distressing for children and parents alike.

Signs and symptoms

 body feels hot; skin can be hot and sweaty, or hot and dry

 temperature is over 37° C (99.5° F) when measured orally (normal temperature for children is 36–36.5° C/96.8–98.6° F)

 red, flushed face; hot hands and feet

 shivery and chilly, although child says he or she feels very hot

 child has no energy, just wants to lie down

Method

Children's temperatures can raise from doing continuous exercise or other strenuous activity, so when taking the temperature for the first time bear that in mind. Check the temperature every half an hour. Let the child lie down somewhere you can see and check up on him or her regularly. Cover the child up, but only with a light cover. If a child shivers, it's the body using another tool at its disposal to lose heat.

The vinegar method for fevers

The old-fashioned European way of dealing with fevers involved vinegar, water and brown paper. Using cloth is an alternative, and we can update and improve the process by adding essential oil. Prepare with the following:

bowl of lukewarm water
2 tablespoons vinegar
lavender – 3 drops.

Put a piece of cloth (or plain, unprinted brown paper) in the bowl, squeeze out, then place it over the child's forehead, making sure that nothing drips into the eyes. When the cloth heats up, remove it and repeat the procedure.

Compress and massage

The following method may help your child sleep.

Add the following essential oils to a bowl of cool (not cold) water:

chamomile roman – 1 drop
lavender – 1 drop
lemon – 1 drop
coriander – 1 drop.

Dip a compress in the water and squeeze out. Place over your child's back for about 5 minutes. Make sure the water isn't cold, but pleasantly cool to the child. Then dry the skin, and massage the back with this oil:

1 teaspoon vegetable oil
rose otto – 2 drops
lavender – 1 drop.

Sponge method

Prepare a bowl of lukewarm (not cold) water, to which you've added a total of 2 drops of essential oil, choosing from the list below. Lavender and eucalyptus radiata are a good mix. Use the water to sponge your child down.

Essential oils that help

lavender
eucalyptus radiata
tea tree
chamomile roman
lemon
spearmint

Other care

Try to make your child as comfortable as possible, and make sure he or she is not wearing too many clothes. A lukewarm bath is cooling, if the child wants to take it, but never force the issue if the child is feeling too unwell. If necessary, sponge your child down on the bed instead. Never use cold water, as this may force the body to work harder and actually raise the temperature. Give your child lots of fluids to drink, including fruit juice to sip. Watch for signs of dehydration (see *Dehydration*).

When to get help

Get medical help if the temperature reaches 39.8° C (103° F), or has been high for longer than 10 hours if there are other symptoms present, or if the child has a convulsion, or is less than 3 months old.

Frostbite

When the temperature is extremely cold, there's a risk of frostbite. It's caused by ice crystals forming in the fluid and tissues of the body, which stop the flow of blood to the affected areas – usually the fingers, toes, nose and ears.

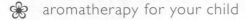
Signs and symptoms

 severe pain in the extremities – including fingers, toes, nose, ears

 initially, skin colour is red, then the affected area becomes numb

 skin may turn a greyish-white to yellow colour, and may blister

 if skin turns black, it is dying and there is the possibility of gangrene setting in

Method

If frostbite occurs, quickly cover the child with as much clothing as possible – especially over the extremities. Do not rub the affected area in an attempt to bring heat into it. Instead, put that area into a bowl of warm (not hot) water, and continue doing so until the skin starts to turn pink. Slowly add hot water to the bowl as needed, to keep the water warm. Essential oils can be added – use 10 drops in a bowl of warm water, choosing from the list below.

If it's the nose that's affected, get any piece of cloth and soak it in warm water, squeeze it out, put 1 drop of geranium on it, and place the cloth over the nose while still warm. Keep repeating until the nose has thawed out and returned to its normal colour. Noses first go red, then gradually lose their colour. Still carry out this warm compress method if the nose is red.

Skin oil

After using the warm water bowl or nose compress method, and the skin is the correct colour again, gently apply a small amount of the following oil:

I tablespoon vegetable oil
geranium – 10 drops
black pepper – 10 drops.

The amount you use will depend upon the area(s) affected. This amount will cover a very large area – you will probably not need to use it all. Use three times a day.

Essential oils that help

geranium
marjoram
black pepper
ginger
helichrysum

When to get help

Get help as soon as possible.

PREVENTION

 If it's cold, wrap your child up very well with waterproof boots or shoes, two pairs of socks and gloves, earmuffs, a hat and a thick scarf that can protect the nose.

Growing pains

Children of any age can suffer with growing pains – some say the pain is 'all over', and not in any particular place; others say the pain is 'in the bones'. Growing pains can be anything from a dull ache to extreme pain, but thankfully they rarely last a long time. Nobody really knows why growing pains happen, although it's fairly clear that in some cases it's because the bones, ligaments and muscles are growing at different rates. Growing pains often occur at night, and can even wake a child up.

Signs and symptoms

 aches in the limbs – source of pain is often uncertain

 muscular soreness

147

pain – between the joints, in the shin and other bones, and other areas of the body

 often felt during the night; or after daytime strenuous physical activity

Method

The first thing to do is rub your hands all over the area the child says is aching, feeling for any swelling or lumps under the skin. If you apply slight pressure around any nearby joint, it will help you decide whether there has been any injury or damage. Ask your child questions to find out if anything happened during the day to cause the pain – did they fall over, for example, or get hurt playing sports? If you find no injury, or reason for the pain, proceed with the growing pains home remedies.

Growing pains can be very distressing for children, who have a great imagination and can get worried about pain that seems to have no cause. Reassure your child that everything is going to be OK, and give lots of sympathy. Massage your child's aching limb(s) and, if it's nighttime, try to stay in the room until they fall asleep. If it's a small child, perhaps they could go in your bed.

Massage oil

Use a small amount of the following oil to massage the arms or legs gently:

1 tablespoon vegetable oil (or calendula-infused oil)
chamomile roman – 3 drops
marjoram – 2 drops.

Use only light pressure, with upward stroking movements, and no pressure at all on the downward strokes.

Apply warmth

Warmth applied to the aching area may bring some relief. This can be done at any time – before or after massaging the limb, for example. Use warm, dry compresses or towels to wrap around painful limbs, or use a warm hot-water bottle (or a wheat bag) to hold against more specific areas.

Warm baths

Warm baths can bring relief to aching limbs. If your child comes home from school complaining of growing pains, run a bath and add the following mix:

1 teaspoon vegetable oil
lavender – 3 drops
marjoram – 1 drop.

The oil will float on the surface of the water. Show your child how to scoop the oil into the palm of the hand and rub it into the painful area of the arm or leg.

A warm bath before bed will help bring a good night's sleep. Refer to the chart on page 9 for the recommended number of drops to use for the different age groups, and choose from the essential oils below.

Essential oils that help

chamomile german
lavender
chamomile roman
calendula-infused oil
marjoram

When to get help

Seek immediate medical help if your child feels pain in the left side of the upper chest. Joint pain and severe arm or leg pain or swelling can be signs of other conditions, such as rheumatism and juvenile arthritis. If the pain continues for longer than 24 hours, consult your physician. Also seek medical help if the pain is accompanied by a high temperature or fever.

Hand, foot and mouth disease

Hand, foot and mouth disease is a viral infection that causes blister-type sores in the mouth, and on the hands and feet. It's more likely to occur during the preschool years, when children routinely put their fingers in their mouths, although children up to around 10 also get it. Infected children spread the virus by touching the blisters, then toys and other objects, or other children. It can also be spread by the child sneezing and coughing, and not washing their hands after going to the toilet. Hand, foot and mouth disease usually lasts around 10 days. It spreads faster in the summer months.

Signs and symptoms

 fever with temperature up to around 39.8° C (103° F), sore throat, feeling unwell, runny nose, cold-type symptoms

 blisters in the mouth; painful sores when they break

 difficulty in eating

 blister-type rash may appear on the hands and feet, and spread to the palms of the hands and soles of the feet and on legs and buttocks

Method

As soon as hand, foot and mouth disease is suspected, apply 1 drop of neat thyme linalol over the glands of the neck, then apply a small amount of vegetable oil over the top. Children with sensitive skin may react to this with reddening of the skin, but this will pass. If your child is old enough to understand the concept of rinsing their mouth and spitting out – and can actually do it – try the mouthwash that follows.

Hand, foot and mouthwash

This wash is for blisters in the mouth, but only if your child is old enough to spit the mixture out. First, mix the following:

30 ml (I ounce) aloe vera juice
30 ml (I ounce) honey water (water with I teaspoon honey mixed in)
cypress – I drop
ravensara – I drop.

Shake the ingredients together in a bottle; the essential oils will still float on the surface. Continue to shake vigorously, then pour through an unbleached, paper coffee-filter into a measuring jug, and rebottle.

Add I teaspoon of the mix to a small wineglass of water and have your child rinse their mouth, making sure they spit it out afterwards. They should not swallow the mouthwash. Repeat as often as possible.

Night-time massage oil

Make up the essential oil mix below, and use 3 drops of the mix, diluted in I teaspoon vegetable oil. Massage over your child's body, avoiding the genital area, every evening before bedtime:

thyme linalol – 5 drops
geranium – 5 drops
niaouli – 5 drops
helichrysum – 5 drops.

Essential oils that help

thyme linalol
lavender
geranium
helichrysum
ravensara
cypress
tea tree
ormenis flower (chamomile maroc)
niaouli
chamomile german
eucalyptus radiata

Other care

Have your child eat bland food, with nothing acidic like oranges and certain fizzy drinks. Give him or her lots of cool drinks, to help with the soreness. Fluid is very helpful at this time. Make honey lollies by adding a spoon of runny honey to melon or other fruit juices, and then freezing. Be careful your child does not share cups or food utensils with other people.

When to get help

Get help if the fever goes over 38.9° C (102° F), or if the blisters do not clear up after 14 days. As this disease has similar symptoms to other conditions, get a proper medical diagnosis.

PREVENTION

 Try to stop your child sucking fingers or thumb.

 Teach your child good hygiene.

Hayfever

Hayfever is an allergic reaction to pollen, and is at its worst during the spring and early summer. In the autumn, weeds such as ragweed can also provoke an attack. Children who are prone to hayfever often come from families where another member has it, or where there is asthma, eczema or psoriasis. Hayfever sufferers may also be sensitive or allergic to certain foods or household products.

Signs and symptoms

   sneezing

   nose congestion; difficulty in breathing properly; runny nose; cold-like symptoms

   red, itchy, sore, watering eyes

   stuffy head

Method

Because hayfever affects people in different ways, you'll need to experiment with the essential oils to see which suits your child best. Surprisingly, perhaps, the flower essential oils can be very helpful in easing the symptoms, and I've found in my practice that both chamomile german and chamomile roman work well, as do the other oils on the 'Essential oils that help' list below.

Tissue method

This method can be used with children over 2 years of age.

Put 1 drop of a hayfever mix on to a tissue, and give it to your child to inhale during the day. Experiment with both mixes, to see which works best.

Hayfever mix 1
Mix together the following. Use 1 drop only, on a tissue:

chamomile roman – 4 drops
lemon – 4 drops
lavender – 2 drops.

Hayfever mix 2
Mix together the following. Use 1 drop only, on a tissue:

geranium – 4 drops
rosemary – 2 drops
eucalyptus radiata – 2 drops.

Evening baths

Make up one of the tissue mixes above, and add to the water in evening baths. Use the amount given below, depending on the age of your child:

under 2 years	1 drop
2–7 years	2 drops
8–11 years	3 drops
over 12 years	4 drops

Diffuser/burner

Diffuse these essential oils in your child's bedroom, as he or she goes to sleep. Do not leave the diffuser there overnight.

helichrysum – 1 drop
lavender – 1 drop

Essential oils that help

lemon
lavender
geranium
neroli
chamomile roman
tangerine
eucalyptus radiata
mandarin
rosemary
grapefruit

Other care

Give your child a small, moist towel or facecloth, secured in a plastic zipped-up bag, to soothe the eyes during the day. Eyedrops may also help. Allergy skin tests can be arranged for children who suffer from hayfever, which may help identify the exact causes of your child's attacks.

PREVENTION

   Keep windows closed when there is a high pollen count.

   Avoid high-pollen areas, or newly mown grass.

   Avoid feather-filled pillows and duvets.

   As dust can make the allergy worse, keep the home as dust-free as possible, with frequent vacuuming and cleaning.

Head lice

Head lice have been a nuisance for human beings, especially small ones, since time began. Lice seem to be an inevitable fact of life, and probably all children will catch them at some time, usually in nursery or primary school. It makes no difference whether the hair is spotlessly clean or dirty, or whether it is short, curly, long or straight. Lice will pass from head to head as children sit close to each other in class, or as they play. They are also passed from person to person if combs and brushes are shared.

The louse is a six-legged insect, smaller than a matchhead but visible to the eye. It bites the scalp and feeds on the blood it sucks out. Then it lays eggs in minuscule white shells, about half an inch from the scalp. When the baby louse comes out, the shell stays attached to the hair shaft. These are called 'nits'. It's often when finding these shells that we become alerted to the fact there are lice in the hair because, unlike dandruff, they cannot be brushed out. The insects themselves are light-sensitive, and very good at hiding.

Problems can occur if the child has been scratching his or her head a lot, and the scalp has become red and irritated, or even infected with bacteria. If the infestation has carried on for a long time, the lymph glands can become enlarged, possibly as an allergic reaction.

Signs and symptoms

 tiny, white, empty shell-cases, attached to the hair shaft, near the scalp

 very small insects on the scalp and in the hair

 itchy scalp, especially at the nape of the neck and behind the ears

Method

Head lice rarely jump on to babies' hair, possibly because there is not so much of it. But even infants can become affected if other members of the family have lice. Because families are in constant close contact, and may share towels, brushes and combs, they are often affected at the same time, so the whole family should be treated at the same time.

It's really important to comb the hair with a fine-toothed comb. This is the only way to get the lice and nits out of the hair. Some of the head lice combs available on the market only collect the insects themselves, leaving the eggs behind. Flea combs for pets are often better because they're often designed for cats, who have very fine hair, and the comb 'teeth' are closer together.

Many of the commercial, chemical preparations should not be used by pregnant women, or infants under 3 years of age. The following mix is safe for pregnant women and for infants if you use only 50 per cent of the amount suggested for others. Only treat small babies if they already have the head lice; it's unlikely they will catch them if other members of the family are treated. Use 3 drops of the mixture below in your usual baby shampoo, and rinse thoroughly.

Head lice scalp oil and rinse

First, mix the ingredients together:

manuka (or kanuka) – 10 drops
tea tree – 10 drops
clove – 5 drops
lavender – 10 drops
thyme linalol – 4 drops
eucalyptus radiata – 5 drops.

Scalp oil
Put 10 drops of the mix above in 1 tablespoon sesame oil, and apply a small amount to the scalp. Do not allow the mixture to go near the eye area, or the nose or ears. Cover the hair with a shower cap and leave for half an hour.

Then, using a fine-toothed comb, gently comb, wiping the comb between each sweep through the hair. Comb the hair an inch section at a time. If the hair is long, you'll need to use clips to separate the hair. When you have combed the whole head, wash the hair with a gentle, baby shampoo. Then, use the rinse below.

Rinse
After shampooing, pour this final rinse through hair, making sure it doesn't get into the eyes, ears, nose or mouth. Use:

120 ml (4 ounces) water
head lice mix (above) – 10 drops.

Shake very well before use.

Scalp-calm

If your child's scalp has become irritated because of the biting, and possible infection, make up the following:

1 teaspoon jojoba oil
chamomile german – 1 drop
lavender – 2 drops.

Apply directly on to the scalp with your fingertips. Gently separate the hair in sections, so you can reach the whole scalp.

Alternative method – the beeswax barrier

An alternative approach to head lice management is to make a barrier between them and their food source – the scalp. Do not attempt this treatment unless you have the exact ingredients listed below, and follow the directions carefully.

You will need a bain-marie (or a pot to go on the cooker), to heat some water, and a heatproof bowl to place in the water. The ingredients are mixed in the bowl. First, melt the beeswax then, while still warm, stir in the castor oil. Keep stirring while you add the essential oils.

8 ml (¼ ounce) natural beeswax (not the white variety)
30 ml (1 ounce) castor oil

While this is still warm, add:

tea tree – 5 drops
lavender – 5 drops
geranium – 5 drops.

Mix together well. When cool enough to apply, take a small amount on your fingertips and dab it on to the scalp – not on the hair. If it does get in some hair, if your ordinary shampoo doesn't remove it, try a dandruff shampoo, or a small amount of bio-degradable washing-up liquid.

Essential oils that help

kanuka
lavender
manuka
eucalyptus radiata
neem
lemongrass
rosemary
thyme linalol
geranium

PREVENTION

 There is not much you can do to prevent your child catching head lice, except to keep long hair tied back, or in a hair band. What you can do is try to prevent it spreading to other members of the family.

 Don't share combs, brushes, towels, pillows or cushions.

 Without being too obvious about it, try to keep those with head lice away from those without.

Headache

See also Migraine.

Most children will complain of headaches now and again, but almost one child in five suffers regularly from headaches, although no cause may be found. Headaches can occur because of overtiredness, stress, toothache, tummy ache, earache, colds and flu. Children may sometimes find it easier to complain of having a headache when there are, in fact, other symptoms they don't want to talk about. Headaches can be symptomatic of more serious disorders, such as high blood pressure, infections, diseases and head injury.

Any headache where there is also neck ache or pain, stiffness, joint pain, when the child cannot bear bright light, or there is fever, vomiting or a feeling of nausea, must be treated as an emergency. Get immediate medical help, as these may be symptoms of meningitis, encephalitis or head injury.

Signs and symptoms

    pain in the head – anything from a mild ache to a throbbing, pounding, severe pain

    pain can be described as located in one particular part of the head, or all over

    in younger children – irritability, tiredness, crying

Method

Before proceeding, ask your child exactly where the pain is. Go through the list of symptoms in 'When to get help' below, asking about each in turn. Take his or her temperature, and ask if there's a sore throat. Be sure also to ask whether he or she had a fall earlier in the day, or the head is hurt in some way. If you are satisfied that your child only has a simple headache, use the following home remedies.

First steps

Have your child lie down, and make a warm drink. Then apply a cool compress to his or her head, made from lavender and peppermint water (see page 18).

Headache mix

First, prepare the headache mix, using:

lavender – 10 drops
chamomile roman – 4 drops
eucalyptus radiata – 10 drops.

This mix can be used in diffusers, or in oil rubs. Use the quantities recommended for your child's age group.

Diffusers
Use 4 drops of the headache mix in diffusers.

Oil rub
Dilute 3 drops of the headache mix in 1 teaspoon vegetable oil. Use a small amount, and rub over the neck and upper back. Also smear a tiny amount over both temples, making sure you avoid the eye area.

Essential oils that help

lavender
chamomile
eucalyptus radiata
lemon
petitgrain
helichrysum
cardamom
myrtle
niaouli

Other care

Fresh air often helps.

When to get help

Get immediate medical assistance if the headache is accompanied by any of the following: neck ache or pain, stiffness, muscle or joint pain, fever, vomiting, a feeling of nausea, or if your child seems sensitive to bright light. Call your doctor if the headache persists.

Heat exhaustion

See also Heatstroke; Sunburn.

When the weather gets very hot, children are at risk of heat exhaustion and, in more serious cases, heatstroke. Read the symptoms in the *Heatstroke* section as well as this, to make sure your child only has heat exhaustion. With heatstroke, you need immediate medical attention.

Signs and symptoms

 dizziness; fainting; fatigue; nausea

 possible raised temperature; perspiration

 possible thirst

 irritability; crying

Heat exhaustion happens when the body overheats due to excessive heat, for example from being in the sun for too long or doing too much exercise. The first thing to do is get the child into a cool, shaded place – preferably inside. Lay the child down, remove most clothing, and get him or her to sip water continuously. If you can add a little salt and sugar to the water, dissolving it well, that will help (see *Dehydration*).

Cooling compress method

Dab a little lavender on the back of your child's neck, on the solar plexus area (above the umbilicus/tummy button), and on both temples – being sure to avoid the eye area.

Put a cool, damp compress or cloth over the back of your child's neck, then cover the body with a light sheet.

Method

If nothing else is available, put a cool, wet cloth on your child's face, and another on the back of his or her neck. Refresh the cloths when they heat up. If the child can sleep, that will help the revival process.

Cooling a body down too rapidly is as bad as not cooling it down at all – someone who cools down too quickly can go into shock. If you use one of the traditional cooling-down methods, like compresses or sponging, use cool water, *never* ice-cold.

Essential oils that help

lavender
petitgrain
eucalyptus radiata

When to get help

Get help if your child's temperature is more than 38.3° C (101° F), or if his or her body has not cooled down after 30 minutes.

PREVENTION

In hot weather

   Make sure your child is always wearing a hat, and the shoulders are covered.

   Keep your child out of the sun as much as possible.

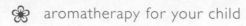

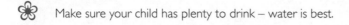 Make sure your child has plenty to drink – water is best.

If running or doing sports

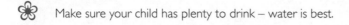 Make sure your child has periods of rest. If you're out in the sun, bring him or her into the shade and the cool.

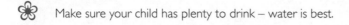 Give your child plenty to drink – water is best.

Heat rash ('prickly heat')

Heat rash is very common amongst babies and small children, although anyone of any age could have it. It happens when the body gets overheated, and sweats too much, causing a blockage in the sweat glands. Babies suffer with it because their sweat glands may not have matured enough to be able to function properly in hot weather.

A heat rash is a collection of tiny blisters, that look like tiny pink or red spots. They can come up anywhere on the body, and can be very itchy. Fortunately, home help can often sort out this problem.

Signs and symptoms

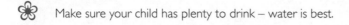 a red rash anywhere on the body, including the face, neck and head

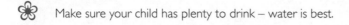 in babies and infants – often in the folds of the skin

Method

As a general rule, try to keep small children's skin dry. On hot days, pat it with a light cotton cloth to absorb sweat. Warm baths are soothing to the skin, but keep the water at just above body-temperature – not too cold, as this may cause shock.

Baths

The temperature of the water should be just above body temperature – not cold.

Essential oil baths
Eucalyptus radiata and lavender are a cooling combination in baths. Make a mix of them, using equal amounts of each. From this, use the following number of drops, for the different age groups:

under 2 years	1 drop
2–7 years	2 drops
8–10 years	3 drops
over 10 years	4 drops

... with baking soda
Add just lavender to the baking soda, mix them well together, then put them in the bath. Don't put them in separately. Use the following amounts, depending on the age of the child:

under 2 years	30 g baking soda	lavender – 1 drop
2–7 years	60g baking soda	lavender – 2 drops
8–10 years	60g baking soda	lavender – 3 drops
over 10 years	100g baking soda	lavender – 4 drops

Essential oils that help

lavender
chamomile roman
eucalyptus radiata

Other care

Keep an eye on babies in warm weather, making sure they wear loose, cool clothing. Put them in cotton, and not in man-made fibres. Open the windows so fresh air can circulate.

When to get help

Get help when all home help has failed – and the rash is still there – or if other symptoms develop (such as vomiting, head pain or continual crying).

PREVENTION

 Keep young babies and infants cool in the heat, with loose, cotton clothing.

 When possible, let the affected skin be exposed to the air.

 Keep the folds of baby's skin dry.

 Keep bottoms dry.

 Don't use baby products that block baby's pores, and avoid those that are mineral-based.

 Try using corn or rice powders instead of talcum powder, making sure your baby inhales none of the powder.

 The condition of the skin can be made worse by certain ingredients in washing powders and liquids that respond to the heat and sweat – enzymes, for example.

Heatstroke

See also Heat exhaustion; Sunburn.

Heatstroke can be life-threatening, and immediate medical help must be sought. Move the child out of the heat and into the shade straight away. While waiting for help to arrive, try to get started on lowering body temperature. With heatstroke, the body's heat regulation system has stopped working and has caused the body temperature to rise. It can happen in extreme heat, when the body fails to adjust to the high temperature, the sweat glands fail to function properly and the body cannot cool itself.

Signs and symptoms

 red-hot skin – could be sweaty or dry

 high temperature

 dizziness; headache; vomiting

 drowsiness – could lead to confusion, and becoming unconscious

 child could have the sensation of being cold, and be shivering

 rapid pulse

 body aches and muscular cramps

Method

If possible, immerse your child's body in cool to tepid water – not cold. Sponge water over the body. Alternatively, stand the child in a lukewarm shower, and gradually reduce the temperature of the water until it's cool – again, not cold. Use any available cool water (even a garden hose, but make the water a very fine spray by applying thumb pressure over the hose exit-hole), and have your child sit down.

Use whatever means you have available to bring your child's body temperature down: wrap them in wet sheets; if you have a fan, use it to cool your child's face. Continue until the temperature is down to 37.2° C (99° F), then cover the child with a dry sheet. Throughout the cooling process, give your child sips of cool water (see *Dehydration*).

Baths	Sponging
Use cool (not cold) water, and add: lavender – 4 drops eucalyptus radiata – 4 drops.	Sponge the body down with cool to tepid water. Put 1 drop of eucalyptus radiata on a sponge, then fill the sponge with water. Start sponging the back of the body first, starting at the back of the neck. Do not sponge the face.

Essential oils that help

lavender
eucalyptus radiata
spearmint
lemon
tangerine
chamomile roman
chamomile german

When to get help

Get help immediately if you suspect your child has heatstroke. In the meantime, while waiting for help to arrive, try to start lowering the child's body temperature.

PREVENTION

In hot weather

   Make sure your child is always wearing a hat, and the shoulders are covered.

   Keep your child out of the sun as much as possible.

   Make sure your child has plenty to drink – water is best.

If running or doing sports

   Make sure your child has periods of rest. If you're out in the sun, bring him or her into the shade, and the cool.

   Give your child plenty to drink – water is best.

Herpes – genital

See also Cold sores ('fever blisters').

The herpes virus exists in two main forms – herpes simplex 1 and 2 – the second of which is basically a blister-like cold sore usually on the genital area. Although it's embarrassing, inconvenient and painful at times, it usually goes in a week or so. Most children with herpes simplex 2 contracted it because their mothers had it and the virus was passed to them during birth. Children can also be infected with herpes by having sexual contact with someone who has it when the virus is active.

Genital herpes usually reappears at the same place on the body where the first contact occurred. The herpes simplex 2 infection is usually thought of as always occurring in the genital area, but I know from clinical experience that people suffer herpes blisters on other parts of their body too – such as the stomach, buttocks, arms and legs.

The first signs of infection are often flu-like symptoms, with fever, aches and pains or headache. These go, and are followed by small blisters around the genital area. Infection is spread through the fluid in the blisters, which usually disappear after a week or so, but infection can re-erupt at any time. With some people this recurrence is frequent, with others it is seldom, and some people only have the initial outbreak and no other in their lifetime. Home treatment aims to reduce the frequency of outbreaks.

Herpes simplex 2 can be triggered by the same things as cold sores – such as heat or stress (*see Cold sores ('fever blisters')* – but because herpes in the genital area can't always be exposed to air, it sometimes takes longer for healing to take effect.

When a child has contracted herpes through their mother, at birth, there may be no visible signs of infection. Such children need to be monitored throughout childhood, and if you are a parent or carer, ask your child's doctor what repercussions are likely for your child.

Signs and symptoms

 tingling, pain or swelling in a genital area, followed by

 blisters – which go in time, but can reappear

Method

Scientific studies have proved that melissa has an effect on herpes. This is one of the most expensive essential oils, and is often difficult to find. Most essential oil suppliers sell a product called 'melissa-type' oil, and not the 'true melissa' you need.

Bathing methods

If the essential oil drops touch an open blister, this may sting temporarily. This will not harm your child, and a small amount of Vaseline over the area will neutralize the effect.

Simple wash
Add 2 drops melissa and 2 drops geranium essential oil to 1 pint water, and bathe the area as often as possible.

Swish the water around before using.

Sitz bath
The sitz bath method involves putting the child's bottom in a large washing-up bowl of water. First, mix the following essential oils:

tea tree – 10 drops
lavender – 6 drops
geranium – 5 drops.

Put 4 drops of the mix in a large plastic bowl of warm water. Then add:

1 tablespoon salt
1 tablespoon bicarbonate of soda

Swish the water around well before your child sits in.

Repeat at least three times a day.

Warm compress method

To help ease the pain, make disposable compresses by using paper kitchen roll. Use a bowl of warm water, adding 5 drops of an essential oil.

Use one of the following:

chamomile german
lemon
geranium
melissa.

Essential oils that help

melissa (but only if 'true melissa')
geranium
thyme linalol
tea tree
manuka
lemon
lavender
chamomile german

Other care

Have your child wear loose clothing in the area of the infection. Growing your own melissa/lemon balm is a good way to get additional help when true melissa is not available – make an infusion of the leaves to bathe the area.

When to get help

Get a proper medical diagnosis.

PREVENTION

 Teach children of all ages to wash their hands after visiting the toilet; and train them to hover above the seat when using the toilet.

 Make sure that sexually active teenagers use condoms.

 If your child has cold sores around his or her mouth or nose (herpes simplex 1), make sure they understand that they should not touch the cold sores and then touch the genital area because this may lead to cross-infection.

While blisters are present

    Pat the area dry – do not rub.

    The child should wash hands after touching sores or blisters.

    Teenagers should not engage in sexual activity while the blisters are present.

Hives (urticaria)

Certain raised white lumps or weals on the skin are known as hives. There are many reasons why they occur, including contact with certain plants, insect bites or stings, and food allergies. Urticaria is a sensitivity to certain substances, which cause the allergic reaction, mostly on the skin, although internal organs can also be affected.

The cause of the hives is often quite obvious – the child has been in contact with a plant, for example, such as nettles or poison ivy, or has been bitten by an insect, like ants, midges, a wasp, bee or hornet. But hives can also appear in response to something consumed, such as shellfish, eggs, nuts, cheese, strawberries, additives or preservatives. Another less obvious cause is an allergic reaction to medication, such as aspirin, penicillin or eyedrops. Some children develop hives as a result of a minor bacterial, viral, fungal or yeast infection – including a strep infection of the nose or throat – or from emotional stress, such as anger or fear. Other children may develop hives in response to the sun and heat, or from exercise, or even from an allergic reaction to the material of the chair they have sat on!

It's important to try to identify what your child is allergic to, so you can avoid further contact. As hives is an allergic reaction, watch your child's face, mouth and tongue, to make sure there is no swelling. If there is, your child may need immediate antihistamine treatment.

Signs and symptoms

 raised weals on the skin – with defined edges that appear raised; white lumps with a red surround; blister-like weals

 weals can be of all sizes and shapes – they are usually confined to one area but, depending on their cause, can disappear, then reappear elsewhere

 stinging, burning sensation at the site of the weals; intense itchiness

 swelling in the area can last up to five days

 headache; feeling unwell; listlessness; cramps

 if the face is swollen, it may indicate angio-neurotic oedema, which can cause the tongue to swell and can be a serious condition

Method

Hives are very irritating, and sleep is one of the best remedies. Gently rub your child's feet. This is calming and may eventually lead to sleep.

Bedtime oil

At bedtime, very gently put a small amount of the following oil over the affected area. Mix the following together:

15 ml (½ ounce) almond oil
chamomile german – 3 drops

lavender – 4 drops
helichrysum – 2 drops
ormenis flower (chamomile maroc) – 2 drops.

Mix the essential oils first, then add to the almond oil.

Hives mix

The following combination of essential oils can be used in compresses and baths:

First, make up the following:

chamomile german – 5 drops
lavender – 5 drops.

From this, use the number of drops recommended in the following methods.

Compress
Use a cool compress to help soothe the area.

Add 2 or 3 drops of the hives mix to the compress water.

Baths
The bath method is more practical when the hives are scattered over different parts of the body.

The temperature of the water should be warm, not hot.

Add 2 or 3 drops of the hives mix above to the bath water.

Adding baking soda to the water will also help, particularly if the hives were caused by an insect bite. Use 1 tablespoon of baking soda per bath.

Essential oils that help

chamomile german
ormenis flower (chamomile maroc)
chamomile roman
helichrysum
lavender

Other care

Calamine lotion can help soothe the skin. Add 4 drops of lavender and 4 drops of chamomile german to 15 ml (1 ounce) calamine lotion.

When to get help

Get immediate medical help if your child has difficulty breathing or if there is any swelling – particularly around the face, mouth or tongue. Antihistamines should be given at the first sign of swelling, or if the hives get worse. Get help if your child is in pain, or if the hives do not disappear after 24 hours.

PREVENTION

 There are so many possible causes of hives there is not much you can do to prevent them on the first occasion. But what you can do is try to prevent further attacks.

 If an insect is the cause, be extra vigilant.

 After the first attack, if there is no obvious plant or insect cause, make a note of all foods your child ate, any medication they took, exercise, stress and weather details. If there is an obvious cause, try to avoid that in the future. If the cause is uncertain, keep your notes for future reference. This way, if a second attack occurs, you may be able to see what same factors were involved.

 If medication is a possible cause, contact your doctor immediately.

Impetigo

Impetigo is a highly contagious skin infection caused by the bacteria *Staphylococcus* and *Streptococcal*. It mainly affects smaller children, and is more common in the summer months. Impetigo is a small rash that can at its worst turn into a pus-filled sore. It usually appears around the mouth or nose first, but can occur anywhere on the body. It's easily spread by contact – if an infected child scratches the area, the bacteria can be transferred to the fingers and spread to other parts of his or her body, or to other children.

Signs and symptoms

 small rash with blister-like spots, usually around the nose or mouth at first – is sometimes mistaken for cold sores

 blisters sometimes filled with pus, becoming open, weeping sores

 sores turn crusty, then a scab forms – and eventually falls off

Method

Wash the affected area thoroughly with soap and water. Use a cloth you can throw away afterwards. Bathing with warm water, and the use of compresses, can give relief. You could use kitchen roll to bathe the area, but use a new piece to dab it dry. Take all measures to prevent cross-infection, including taking care to wash your own hands with anti-bacterial soap after carrying out home-care

Compress method

To one dessertspoon of melissa or lavender hydrolat/water, add 1 drop of chamomile german. Use to soak the compress, and apply over the affected area.

Impetigo mix

Use the following mix in the tea-dab and oil methods below. First, mix these essential oils:

ravensara – 15 drops
thyme linalol – 10 drops
tea tree – 15 drops
manuka – 10 drops (if not available, substitute an extra 10 drops of tea tree).

Tea-dab
After bathing, dab over the area with the following tea.

Use the whole mix above in 60 ml (2 ounces) water. See page 54 for how to make the tea.

Lavender and melissa hydrolats are very useful when used to bathe affected areas. If you have these hydrolats, use them instead of water in the above tea.

Oil
Use the whole mix above in 8 ml ($^1/_4$ ounce) sesame oil.

Blend well, and apply a small amount on affected areas only.

Use between bathing.

Essential oils that help

ravensara
thyme linalol
manuka
tea tree
lavender
niaouli
chamomile german

Other care

See 'Prevention' below.

When to get help

If you suspect impetigo, see your doctor for a firm diagnosis.

 Avoid contact with children who have the infection.

If your child is infected

 Keep fingernails short to prevent the spread of the infection.

 The child, and all other members of the family, should wash with anti-bacterial soap.

 Take measures to stop the itching.

 Make sure the child uses separate facecloths, towels and linen.

 Change pillowcases every day, to prevent the infection spreading to other parts of the face.

Although it is common to send infected children to school with their impetigo covered up, this may not always stop infection spreading. It may be advisable to keep your child off school if they have the infection, for the sake of the other children in the class. Please check with your child's school for their policy on contagious infections.

Influenza ('flu')

The term 'flu' is given to various strains of the same airborne influenza virus, which all cause more or less the same type of symptoms. It can last anything from a day to two weeks, depending on the strain of the virus. Each strain causes a particular set of symptoms, with some causing more sore throats, for example, while others will seem to have more effect on the muscles. They will all pass eventually, but home treatment with essential oils will cut down the time of suffering and aid a full recovery.

Signs and symptoms

 muscular aches and pains

 headache

 sore throat; cough

 high temperature and fever; but often
also shivering and feeling cold

 red eyes; runny nose

 weakness; tiredness; irritability; crying

in some cases – vomiting; diarrhoea

Method

If one member of the household has flu, diffuse or spray
anti-viral essential oils in the atmosphere, to try and keep
cross-infection down.

**Children under
3 years**

Apply the following mix
to the upper chest and
back:

1 teaspoon almond oil
thyme linalol – 1 drop
ravensara – 2 drops.

Children over 4 years

Only use this method if you have these essential oils available:

thyme linalol (no other type of thyme can be substituted)
ravensara.

First open both bottles of oil. Put 1 drop of thyme linalol in the palm of one hand, and add 1 drop of ravensara to it. Rub your hands together and rub over your child's back. Then immediately smooth over the same area using between $1/4$ and $1/2$ teaspoon vegetable oil. Do the same thing on the child's upper chest.

This is one of the few times the professional method of using essential oils directly on the skin is recommended for home use, but make sure you only use the essential oils listed above.

Body massage

Make a massage oil by mixing:

8 ml ($1/4$ ounce) almond oil
thyme linalol – 5 drops
ravensara – 5 drops.

Use 1 teaspoon of the above mix to massage the arms and legs, as well as the neck, back and front. Avoid the genital area.

Night-time methods

Diffuser/spray
Before your child goes to sleep, diffuse 2 drops from the following essential oil recipe in their room:

red thyme – 2 drops
oregano – 2 drops
cinnamon – 2 drops
clove – 2 drops.

If using a diffuser, make sure it is not left in the child's room overnight.

Essential oils that help

ravensara
thyme linalol
eucalyptus radiata
niaouli

Other care

Children get bored and miserable when they have flu, so keep him or her near you during the day by making up a bed on the sofa. What they need most is kind, loving attention – and plenty of rest. Try to reduce any fever with the compress method. Avoid giving milk products, as they increase the mucus within the body. Give small drinks of pure fruit juice, and lots of water.

When to get help

Get medical advice if your child is asthmatic, diabetic or has a weakened immune system. The symptoms of flu are similar to those of other infections and diseases, so watch to make sure your child does not develop a rash – if so, consult your doctor immediately. Also get medical help if your child complains of earache, if the cough gets worse or if the temperature does not go down after 36 hours.

PREVENTION

Flu is all too easy to catch and there's not much you can do to prevent it. But you can try to stop it spreading to other members of the family.

 If other members of the family are at home, keep a child with flu in bed and isolated from other people.

 Dispose of used tissues in a closed bin immediately after use.

Ingrowing toenails

When the side of a toenail becomes embedded in the surrounding tissue, instead of growing straight outwards, it is said to be ingrowing. A nail might grow into the tissue because of a natural curve, or more likely because ill-fitting shoes have forced it in that direction. Shoes that are too narrow across the toes are often to blame.

Signs and symptoms

 usually affects the big toe

 the area around the ingrowing toenail is very sore, and particularly painful when walking

 tissue around the ingrowing toenail is red and swollen

 area around the nail can become infected

Method

Footbath

Soaking the toes in water softens the nails – adding the following essential oils to the water may help to avoid the area becoming infected. Soak the affected area at least twice a day. To a footbath, add:

lavender – 2 drops
tea tree – 2 drops
1 teaspoon salt
1 teaspoon Epsom salts
1 teaspoon baking soda.

Essential oils that help

lavender
tea tree
helichrysum
ravensara
chamomile roman

Other care

Get your child to wear open-toed shoes whenever possible, and to go barefoot or in socks when at home.

To relieve the pain and prevent infection

Put I drop of the following essential oil mix around the toe area, twice a day:

lavender – 5 drops
tea tree – 5 drops.

When to get help

A doctor or chiropodist will usually be able to remove the embedded section of nail and dress the toe, although surgery is sometimes required. Even after a toenail has been correctly cut, it can still become more inflamed. If your child develops a temperature, or if you see any sign of a white mass under the nail, get medical attention because there could be an infection. When you first suspect your child might have an ingrowing toenail, and even if it's not very painful, get medical advice. It's important to deal with this problem now, to prevent difficulties in later life.

PREVENTION

 Ingrowing toenails are often an ongoing problem, so check on the nail as it grows, and take prompt action if it happens again.

 Make sure your child's shoes are not too tight – widthways, as well as lengthways.

Laryngitis

Laryngitis is a mild inflammation of the larynx, vocal cords and voice box. It can last up to a week and is not generally serious except potentially for babies and small children. Laryngitis can be caused by viral and bacterial infection, allergy, irritation from a smoky atmosphere, or by using the voice too much. Professional singers are prone to laryngitis, as are people who shout loudly at football matches. Laryngitis is more common during the autumn and winter months, when many cold and flu viruses seem to be around.

Signs and symptoms

 sore throat; hoarse voice

 difficulty in swallowing; breathing difficulties

 dry cough

 possibly – fever; tiredness; generally feeling unwell

 baby will sound hoarse when it cries, with possible voice loss

 larynx can become swollen and obstruct the airways of smaller infants; can lead to croup

Method

Laryngitis is a common problem, and people have found many natural ways to help ease the symptoms. An opera singer once told me that she and her colleagues relied on tinned peaches in syrup – which they either ate, or put through a blender and sipped all day. Apparently it worked wonderfully.

Keeping the air moist is very helpful, and this can be done using a humidifier, room spray or bowls of steaming water. Baths and showers also provide moist air for a short time. Essential oils

185

can be used in all these methods. See page 8 for directions on how to prepare the different methods; the list on page 27 for the number of drops of essential oil to use for children of different ages; and the 'Essential oils that help' or the laryngitis mix given below.

Laryngitis mix

The following mix can be used in the 'Soothing oil mix' and 'Cool compress' method below. Follow the directions in each box. First mix together:

chamomile german – 5 drops
ravensara – 5 drops
helichrysum – 2 drops.

Soothing oil mix
Add the laryngitis mix above to:

30 ml (1 ounce) vegetable oil.

Use a small amount each time. Gently apply over the front of the neck.

Cool compress
Add 3 drops of the laryngitis mix above to a small bowl of cool (not cold) water. Soak a compress in the water, squeeze out and apply over the front of the neck.

Laryngitis tea

Only a small amount of this tea is used each time.

Put three lemons, and a handful of fresh mint if you have it, into a teapot and cover with 1/2 pint boiling water. Add 1 tablespoon honey, and stir before replacing the lid. Leave to cool. Then add 1 drop of lemon essential oil, stir again, and pour through an unbleached paper coffee-filter.

Children over 5 can sip 1 tablespoon of the tea in a glass of warm water.

Essential oils that help

ravensara
chamomile german
ginger
thyme linalol
eucalyptus radiata
helichrysum
cajuput
geranium

Other care

Give your child plenty of soothing, warm (but not hot) drinks, such as warm water and honey; warm water, honey and lemon; or warm water and fruit juice. To allow the throat inflammation to calm down, stop your child from shouting or talking a lot, as that will only make the hoarse voice worse. Let fresh air into the home, and keep the atmosphere moist.

When to get help

Babies and infants with laryngitis need to be closely watched, to make sure the larynx does not become swollen and obstruct the airways, in which case, immediate medical attention must be sought. If the laryngitis develops into croup (see *Croup*), see your doctor as soon as possible. Also seek medical advice if your child develops a high temperature, or if you suspect there may be an infection other than laryngitis.

Lyme disease

Lyme disease is caused by a micro-organism carried by a tick that usually lives on deer. Infection can occur if a person is bitten by one of these deer ticks, although the disease is not transmitted unless the tick has remained attached to the skin for around 24 hours. The ticks live in grassy and woodland areas, and are more active during the summer. It's often difficult to realize that infection has occurred because the ticks are so small and easily overlooked that the bite is not felt, and a rash does not always develop. Lyme disease was only recognized as a specific condition in 1975. A blood test is needed to get a positive diagnosis.

Signs and symptoms

 when bitten, a circular red rash appears, with a distinct spot in the middle

 the rash clears, leaving a circular mark

 in the weeks following the bite, a rash could occur on other parts of the body

 flu-like symptoms, including fever, headache, muscle ache and pain, listlessness, tiredness and irritability

 arthritis-like symptoms can develop over time – with swollen and painful joints

 in the worst cases – central nervous system is affected, with numbness, paralysis and heart problems

Method

Lyme disease is a very serious condition and requires a proper diagnosis and medical treatment. Essential oils can help as a deterrent – to stop the ticks from coming near your child. Also, after being bitten, if you are camping and far away from medical facilities, essential oils can be used as emergency treatment until you can get medical help.

Deterrent clothing spray

If you are going into an area where deer live and the tick may be present, prepare the following mix and take it with you, stored in a spray bottle. Use to spray clothing – especially around the neckline, cuffs, the hems of skirts or bottoms of trouser legs, on shoes, socks and the outside of hats. Allow to dry, then repeat.

In a small bowl, first mix the following:

citronella – 30 drops
lemongrass – 30 drops
eucalyptus radiata – 20 drops
peppermint – 10 drops
niaouli – 10 drops.

Then add 8 ml ($^1/4$ ounce) neem oil – if you can get it (neem comes from India – ask in Indian shops).

Next, pour 250 ml (8 ounces) hot water on to the mix, and put a plate over the bowl so the condensed steam-water is caught in the mix when the water cools.

Leave it to stand for at least 48 hours.

Finally, strain the mix through a paper coffee-filter, and bottle.

Neat oils – clothing deterrent mix

Make up a mix, using the same essential oils listed in the clothing spray above.

Put 1 or 2 drops on socks, trouser bottoms, hems, shirt cuffs and collars, and around hat brims. Some essential oils may mark clothing; apply on areas which do not touch skin.

Use on the clothing of children over 7 years.

For children under 7, use neat niaouli and eucalyptus radiata essential oil, in the same method as above. An alternative deterrent is lavender oil, but try to avoid that if you regularly use it to help your child to sleep.

Deterrent body massage oil

This body massage may help prevent your child being bitten. It can be used during the night or in the day. It can also be used on children who have already been bitten. Rub the oil all over the body. This is enough for several applications. Mix together:

1 tablespoon vegetable oil
niaouli – 2 drops
lavender – 3 drops.

Emergency care

If your child has been bitten and you are camping far from medical help, put a couple of neat drops of whatever essential oil you have with you directly on the bite, before extracting the tick with tweezers.

Then wash the bite thoroughly with soap and water, and put 1 drop of neat lavender or thyme linalol directly on the bite.

Try to get help as soon as possible.

In the meantime, repeat the wash and neat essential oil application at least once a day, and use the body massage method on the child as well.

Using essential oils as insect deterrents has become very popular. The list below contains essential oils that are suitable for use on children's clothing. As these will be used while hiking or camping, I assume the child will not be wearing any expensive, delicate clothing, as some of these essential oils may leave a mark on the material.

Essential oils that help

to deter ticks
lavender
eucalyptus radiata
niaouli
peppermint
thyme linalol
lemongrass
citronella
palmarosa

to ease tick bite
thyme linalol
niaouli
eucalyptus radiata
lavender

with the rash
chamomile german
lavender

When to get help

Call a doctor immediately if you suspect that your child has been bitten, as early treatment prevents damage in later life.

PREVENTION

Prevention is much better than cure. Take precautions if your child is playing in long grass or woods where deer live.

 Have your child wear long sleeves and trousers – and tuck trouser legs into socks. Put a hat on your child, and see that he or she wears light-coloured clothing.

 Spray clothing with an insect deterrent. Be careful if using preparations that contain deet.

 Check your child for any tiny ticks – look in the hairlines, as well as more obvious places.

 If you see a tick, remove it very carefully with tweezers and apply disinfectant to the area. To make a correct diagnosis easier, take the tick with you to the doctor.

 If you take a pet into the area, check them for ticks also.

Measles (rubeola)

Measles is a highly contagious, airborne, viral infection, and is spread through coughing and sneezing. After exposure to the virus, the incubation period is around 10–14 days. Despite large-scale imunization, cases do still occur. Most affected children go through the infection with no bad side effects, but measles is potentially very dangerous because it makes a child vulnerable to other infections – such as bronchitis and pneumonia, and to ear infections, which can lead to deafness.

Signs and symptoms

 begins with cold-like symptoms: runny nose, cough, fever, listlessness

 small red spots with white centres, on the tissue lining the inside of the mouth

 red itchy rash appears two to four days after the spots in the mouth – starts at the forehead, spreads over the face, neck, behind the ears, then over the tummy and to other areas of the body

 red, sore eyes, which are sensitive to bright light

 respiratory difficulties

 possibly – abdominal pain, vomiting, diarrhoea

Method

There are many approaches to aromatherapy measles management, including: baths and sponging to soothe the rash and aid recovery, the humidifier method for coughs that do not ease, rest for the body, compresses for sore eyes, and diffusers and other room methods to prevent the infection from spreading.

Soothing baths

Oat bath
Put a handful of raw oats or oatmeal in a piece of material, and add to it:

chamomile german –
4 drops
lavender – 4 drops
ravensara – 4 drops.

Tie the bundle securely, then attach it to the bath tap, so the water can run through the bundle before reaching the bath.

Oil bath
Put 1 tablespoon sea salt in the bath water.

Then dilute the following essential oils in 1 teaspoon vegetable oil:

lavender – 1 drop
bergamot – 2 drops
tea tree – 3 drops.

Also add to the bath.

Swish the water around well before the child gets in.

Bicarbonate of soda bath
Mix the following essential oils in 100g bicarbonate of soda:

lavender – 2 drops
chamomile german –
1 drop
geranium – 4 drops.

Mix the essential oils in thoroughly with a spoon. Then add to the bath water.

Sponging method

First, mix the following:

bergamot – 5 drops
chamomile german –
5 drops
lavender – 5 drops.

Use 5 drops for each sponge-down to help reduce fever. Put tepid or warm (not hot) water in a small bowl and add 5 drops of the essential oil mix. Swish the water around, then soak a sponge or facecloth in it, squeeze it out, and use to sponge down the whole of your child's body – avoiding the face and genital area.

Humidifier

If your child has a cough that does not ease, use essential oils from the list below in humidifiers and steaming baths:

niaouli
ravensara
cajuput

Rest

To help the child get a good night's sleep, put 1 or 2 drops of chamomile roman or lavender on a corner of his or her pillow – on the underside, away from eyes.

If neither of these helps, try neroli essential oil, which is sometimes effective when the others are not.

Eye compress

If your child's eyes are sore, place a cool wet cloth over them.

You could also make a chamomile roman tea, following the instructions on page 54, or a chamomile hydrolat, and use one of them for the compress water. Make sure you squeeze the compress out well, and that your child keeps his or her eyes closed.

Preventative atmosphere

To help prevent the spread of infection, use the vaporizer, diffuser or water-spray method (see page 15). Mix the following essential oils:

bergamot – 10 drops
ravensara – 20 drops
geranium – 10 drops.

Use 4–6 drops each time.

If you do not have these essential oils, use any from the list below.

Essential oils that help

chamomile german
lavender
niaouli
ravensara
thyme linalol
cajuput
eucalyptus radiata
tea tree
bergamot

Other care

Your child must stay in bed, and be kept away from other children – even if they have been immunized. Adults can also catch measles and, as with many other so-called 'childhood' diseases, it can be far worse for adults. Make sure you take all possible precautions to avoid catching the infection yourself.

When to get help

If you suspect measles, consult your child's doctor immediately. If your child recovers from measles and then gets worse again, possibly with an earache, go back to your doctor. Inform your child's school that they have measles, so other parents can be told to watch for signs and symptoms in their children.

PREVENTION

   Although immunization has certainly stopped the spread of this potentially dangerous infection, doubts have been raised as to the total safety of the vaccine.

If your child is allergic to eggs tell your doctor, because the measles vaccine is developed on eggs, and this may cause a reaction in your child.

Menarche – menstrual problems

Menarche is the onset of the menstrual cycle. The average age at which girls start their periods is 11–13, but do bear in mind that some girls start as early as 8 while others find themselves waiting until they're 17 or 18.

Signs and symptoms

 uterine cramps

 backache

 flow can be light or heavy – the first flow can be very dark

Method

It's important to prepare your daughter for the onset of menarche, by giving her sanitary towels and showing her how to use them, and by telling her it will start unexpectedly, with a feeling of wetness or discomfort.

Girls often feel embarrassed about menstruation and don't want fathers or brothers to know they've started. Be sensitive to your daughter's wishes about this, because if you betray her trust on this important occasion she may be less inclined to confide in you during her later teens – perhaps over issues you may need to know about.

Tummy rub

Geranium essential oil is a blessing for women of all ages, as it is a great help in dealing with cramps and blood-flow problems.

Put 4 drops of neat geranium oil on the tummy, over the uterine area, and spread it around. Then cover this area with a small amount of vegetable oil.

Let your daughter sit and rest with something warm over the area. If you use a hot-water bottle, use warm (not hot) water; or use the type of bag that can be heated in a microwave.

Warm baths

The following essential oil bath can help with all the symptoms of menstruation, plus lessen any anxiety your daughter may be feeling. Mix together:

1 teaspoon vegetable oil
geranium – 3 drops
bergamot – 1 drop
lavender – 2 drops.

Pour the mixture into the bath, as the warm water is running. Tell your daughter that if she find globules of oil floating on the water, scoop them into her hand and rub the oil into her skin, over the tummy. If her breasts are sore, she can massage the floating oil into them as well.

Essential oils that help

geranium
rose
lavender
chamomile roman
helichrysum

When to get help

Medical help is not usually required when girls start menstruating. However, you should seek advice if your daughter's cramps are so bad she can't move without pain; if she has pain urinating or defaecating; or if she has severe premenstrual syndrome (PMS).

Meningitis

Meningitis is caused by several different types of bacteria and virus, and leads to inflammation of the lining of the brain (meninges). It is spread by an infected person sneezing, coughing or kissing, and by poor hygiene or unsanitary water.

The bacterial types of meningitis can be life-threatening if not detected early enough, while the viral types are much less severe. Early diagnosis is the key to treating meningitis and, if you have any suspicion your child has this infection, do not wait for help, but take your child straight away to the nearest medical facility and demand that they are seen immediately.

The difficulty with meningitis is that the early symptoms are very similar to those for flu. This can confuse doctors, as well as parents. The symptoms of both bacterial and viral meningitis are similar to begin with, and the illness can develop over a couple of days. However, in serious cases there can come a point when the child suddenly gets worse.

If your child has symptoms of meningitis, it's important to find out which type it is, as the viral types of meningitis are much more common – and much less dangerous – than the bacterial type. If you suspect meningitis, go to the nearest hospital and have tests to ascertain which type your child has. Antibiotics cannot fight viral meningitis, and treatment for this type usually just consists of good nursing care.

Bacterial meningitis is the one everyone worries about. There are two types: meningococcal and pneumococcal. The first symptoms will usually appear 2–10 days after infection. Most children will make a full recovery if diagnosis and treatment are given early; however, bacterial meningitis can lead to deafness, brain damage or even death. Children of all ages are at risk, including newborn babies.

The symptom lists below refer to the most usual symptoms. An affected child might just have one of these symptoms, or many of them.

Signs and symptoms in babies

     fever; yet the hands and feet might feel cold and look blue

     blank, staring expression

     may refuse food, or vomit

     may be difficult to wake up; baby has no energy

     fontanelle – the soft spot on the top of the skull – may feel tense, or bulge

     makes strange noises – whimpering, or a high-pitched moan

     does not like to be picked up

     neck retraction – the head is pushing backwards; often with arched back

     skin is pale or blotchy

Signs and symptoms in children

     symptoms may seem similar to those of flu

     stiff neck

     high temperature; fever

     severe headache

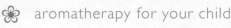

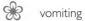 vomiting

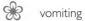 pain in joints or muscles

 dislike of bright light

 seizure

 drowsiness; lethargy

 small purplish-red rash that can still be seen when a glass is pressed against it; more rashes appear
– anywhere on the body

Method

One of the symptoms of meningitis is neck pain. Don't just ask your child if their neck hurts: they are likely to say yes even if they only have flu. Gently take your child's head in your hands and try to move it. First move it upwards, then downwards, then to one side, then the other. If your child now says the neck hurts, or if the neck cannot move, then meningitis may be present.

Another symptom of meningitis is joint or muscle pain. If a child complains of 'pains in the leg' (or a smaller child might volunteer 'leg hurt'), this might indicate meningitis. Sensitivity to light is a classic symptom of meningitis – bring a table lamp to your child, or use a torch if nothing else is available, and watch your child's reaction closely. They may screw up their eyes or whimper, or pull away. Babies with meningitis have the symptom of disliking being picked up or handled by you. This is very unusual for a baby, especially if they are ill with something less severe than meningitis. Take this symptom seriously. Also, with a baby, feel the top of their head in the fontanelle region – if it bulges or feels hard, this is a classic symptom of meningitis.

The characteristic rash that accompanies some forms of meningitis – particularly the bacterial meningococcal strain – shows that blood poisoning (septicaemia) has taken place. If you get a clear glass and press it against a meningitis rash, it stays clearly visible through the glass. With most other rashes, when you press a glass against it, it will temporarily fade.

Meningitis is a life-threatening disease and requires immediate medical treatment. Although there are essential oils with anti-bacterial and anti-viral properties it is only appropriate at this time to use essential oils to soothe the child, and to help with some of the symptoms. Choose from the methods on pages 9–17, using the number of drops recommended for the different age groups.

The viral types of meningitis are treated with good nursing care – and this is where essential oils can really help. Use essential oils in baths, and in hand and foot massages. Don't massage the whole body. Room sprays are useful at this time, as they can uplift a sick child, cheering them up slightly, and offer protection against cross-infection. Essential oils used in the water-spray method, over your child's bed-linen, can help freshen up that area. A favourite essential oil combination with children, which would help cheer them up at this time, consists of equal parts geranium and orange.

Essential oils that help

The following essential oils can be used alongside conventional medical treatment, and used to help lessen the symptoms of meningitis. For the appropriate dosage – the number of drops to use – see page 27.

chamomile roman
chamomile german
lavender
ormenis flower (chamomile maroc)
cardamom
palmarosa
ravensara
niaouli

Other care

Give your child plenty of fluid to drink, especially water.

When to get help

Always get immediate emergency help if you suspect meningitis.

PREVENTION

 Speak to your physician about immunization. There are vaccines for some forms of meningitis, including haemophilus influenzae type b (Hib).

 Be especially vigilant if your child has recently had another type of illness – such as mumps, a throat infection or flu – as meningitis sometimes erupts after having these.

 If meningitis has been diagnosed in other local children, keep your child away from all children as much as possible.

 If your child has meningitis, inform the school straight away, so other parents can be warned to look for symptoms in their children.

Migraine

A migraine is an attack of severe pain and continual ache in the head. There are different types of migraine – some cause nausea and sickness or make a child shield their eyes from the light, while others do not. Migraine might run in the family, or not. Each individual has different 'triggers' – it may be stress or anxiety, computer overuse, perfumes, pollutants, bright lights, being in a stuffy atmosphere, or eating a food they are allergic to (classic culprits are cheese, the caffeine in milkshakes, chocolate, oranges, tomatoes, and spicy foods). Each child will have an individual 'profile' of migraine causes, and an individual symptom 'profile' that may include some or all of those below.

Signs and symptoms

 head pain and ache – often over one eye and down one side of the face

 disturbed vision; eye ache

 seeing strange colours around objects, like auras

 pale skin tone

 abdominal pain; neck ache

 tingling and other unusual sensations in the body

numb feeling in the head and face

abnormal sense of smell – either loss of smell or heightened smell

Method

Cold compresses

Cold compresses can give some relief. Put 1 pint of cold water in a small bowl and add:

grapefruit – 3 drops
lavender – 2 drops

Put a light cloth in the bowl, squeeze out well, and place on the back of your child's neck, or on the forehead – making sure the compress is well squeezed out.

Put the unused compress water in the refrigerator to keep cool, and use it to refresh the compress during the migraine attack.

General migraine body massage

First, blend the following essential oils:

chamomile roman – 5 drops
grapefruit – 10 drops
peppermint – 5 drops
rosemary – 3 drops.

If your child is under 7 dilute the above in 120 ml (4 ounces) vegetable oil

If your child over 8 dilute in 40 ml (1 ½ ounces) vegetable oil

Use a small amount of the diluted oil in a massage – at least 15 minutes, once a week. Take the phone off the hook, and have your child lie on their front. Gently massage the back, shoulders, legs and arms, always working towards the direction of the heart.

Stress migraine body massage

This massage oil is helpful if your child's migraine is brought on by stress. Use equal amounts of the essential oils of:

neroli
petitgrain.

See page 27 for the appropriate number of drops of essential oil to use for the age of your child. Dilute the appropriate number of drops of essential oil in vegetable oil.

Use a small amount of diluted oil in a body massage – at least 15 minutes, once or twice a week. Take the phone off the hook, and have your child lie on his or her front. Gently massage the back, shoulders, legs and arms, always working towards the heart.

Regular gentle massage will help to keep your child less stressed, and also introduce a parent's loving touch.

Nausea tummy rub

If your child suffers from nausea and sickness during a migraine attack, prepare the essential oil mix as for the 'General migraine body massage' above and, instead of massaging the whole body, you could just rub a little of the diluted oil over your child's abdomen, and the back of the neck.

Essential oils that help

grapefruit
lavender
chamomile roman
neroli
petitgrain
marjoram
peppermint
rosemary

Other care

Lie your child down on a bed or sofa, pull the curtains to darken the room, making sure there is a window open, in order to air the room. Your child may feel sick, so put a bucket nearby for him or her to be sick into – having to run to the bathroom to be sick will only make your child feel worse.

Give your child plenty of liquids – in some children, grapefruit juice has been helpful in lessening the severity of the attack. Make sure your child has eaten – migraine often comes on if a child has skipped lunch or breakfast. Give something light to eat – even if your child feels sick and says he or she doesn't want anything, it may make him or her feel better. Then your child needs quiet, rest and sleep.

When to get help

See your doctor if your child complains of stomach pains or has recurring migraine attacks.

PREVENTION

 Keep a diary to try and find out what causes the migraine. Write down all foods and drinks consumed prior to the attack, what subjects were coming up on your child's school timetable, who came to visit your home, and where your child visited. Try to eliminate the triggers. It may be that certain people or places make your child stressed or anxious. Your child may be having an allergic reaction to a chemical or pollutant in the atmosphere. Or did he or she spend too long watching TV, or on the computer? Write everything that happens on the day of the attack, so you can compare notes if it happens again. There are so many possible causes of migraine, all you can do is try to narrow them down. In this way, you may be able to identify triggers to your child's migraine, and avoid them in the future.

Mononucleosis (mono – 'kissing disease')

Mono is a common viral infection caused by the Epstein-Barr virus, a member of the herpes family. It's often transmitted by mouth contact and saliva, which is why it's called 'the kissing disease' and why teenagers are the group that is usually affected. However, mono can also be caught by younger children, by breathing in infected droplets in the air. The symptoms appear around two weeks after infection, and the condition usually clears up after a week or so.

Signs and symptoms

 'flu-like symptoms; aches and pains; generally feeling unwell

 fatigue and overwhelming tiredness

 swollen lymph nodes/glands in the neck

sore throat; enlarged tonsils covered with mucus

 high temperature

Method

Back, chest and throat oil

The following oil can be rubbed over your child's back, chest and throat. Mix the essential oils first, then add to the vegetable oil.

Use a small amount each time.

1 tablespoon vegetable oil
tea tree – 10 drops
lemon – 5 drops
eucalyptus radiata – 10 drops
ravensara – 6 drops.

Sore throat gargle mix

Only use this method if your child is old enough to spit the water out after the gargle. It will help ease a sore throat.

First, using the 'tea' method (outlined on page 54), make a 'tea' with lemon and geranium essential oil.

For the gargle – put the following in a small glass of water:

1 teaspoon lemon and geranium 'tea'
1/2 teaspoon salt
1 teaspoon vinegar.

Stir well, and have your child gargle with this, making sure he or she spits it out afterwards. Repeat three times a day.

Warm baths

Warm baths will help make your child feel better. Add 4 drops of the following mix to 1 teaspoon vegetable oil, and add to the bath water:

ravensara – 3 drops
mandarin – 5 drops.

This is enough for two baths.

Diffuser

To help your child sleep well, use the following essential oils in a diffuser in your child's bedroom, as he or she goes to sleep:

lavender – 2 drops
chamomile roman – 1 drop
mandarin – 3 drops.

Don't leave the diffuser in the room overnight.

Essential oils that help

lavender
ravensara
niaouli
cajuput
chamomile roman

Other care

Give your child plenty of fluid. He or she should do no strenuous exercise, and must rest.

When to get help

Contact your doctor if the young person or child develops a high fever; has breathing difficulties; or if the tiredness and weakness continues after the infection has passed.

PREVENTION

 Avoid contact with infected persons.

If your child has mono

 Keep your child isolated from other members of the household.

 Dispose of all mucus-laden tissues in a closed bin immediately after use.

 Teach your child to cough directly into a tissue, and dispose of it by flushing it down the toilet.

Motion sickness

Motion sickness can result from travelling in cars, boats, trains, planes and amusement-park rides, and even from playground swings. Travel by car is the most common cause of motion sickness, and can be made worse for sensitive children by general road pollution or leakages of fuel fumes from the vehicle itself.

Motion sickness is caused by the delicate mechanism in the inner ear and the fluids contained in it, becoming out of balance by repeated movement of the head and body. Fast-moving, conflicting messages being received from the eyes to the brain don't help.

In some children, the very thought of having to travel makes them tense and anxious, and they begin to get some of the symptoms of motion sickness before they've even stepped outside the front door!

Signs and symptoms

 vomiting; feeling unwell; feeling faint; dizziness; perspiration

 drowsiness; yawning; breathing more heavily

cold, clammy feel to the skin, or unusual pallor to skin

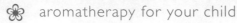 in some cases, earache

Method

If the child vomits, give some liquid to make sure he or she doesn't get dehydrated.

Teas

These methods can only be used on children over 2 years of age. Make up one of the following teas beforehand, cool and bottle, and take it with you. Have the child sip it slowly during the journey.

Make tea with fresh peppermint herb and root ginger. Slice a small piece of fresh ginger and some pieces of fresh mint. Add boiling water, cover, and leave to brew for at least 10 minutes. Bottle when cold.

Make tea using one peppermint and one ginger teabag. Cover and leave to brew for 10 minutes. Bottle when cold.

To make a tea using essential oils, follow the directions on page 54, and use:

peppermint – 1 drop
ginger – 1 drop.

Use 1 tablespoon of the finished tea, added to 30 ml (1 ounce) water. No more than 75 ml (3 ounces) should be consumed during the journey.

Babies

Exclude peppermint from blends for babies under 2 years of age, and only use the vehicle tissue method.

Put 1 drop of the 'Motion sickness mix' on a tissue and tuck somewhere in the travel vehicle.

Give the baby sips of cooled, boiled water during the journey.

Motion sickness mix

Mix together:

ginger – 10 drops
peppermint – 4 drops
eucalyptus radiata – 2 drops
coriander – 2 drops.

Dilute 2 drops of the mixture in 1 teaspoon vegetable oil, and rub a small amount over the child's back and abdomen before the journey starts.

Other

Put 1 drop of the 'Motion sickness mix' on a tissue and tuck it down the seat behind the child.

Put 4 drops of ginger oil on a tissue and let your child sniff it, as required.

Flying anxiety

Before travelling
For the younger child, add 1 drop of lavender and 1 drop of geranium to a small amount of vegetable oil, and put it in the bath. It will float, and can be collected in the hands and massaged into the child's skin, under the water. Older children can massage it in for themselves.

During the flight
Take with you a preprepared mix of 5 drops each of chamomile, lavender and geranium, diluted in 30 ml (1 ounce) vegetable oil. Younger children will allow you to massage a little of this into their feet, while for older children place 2 drops of lavender on to a tissue and place it behind them, on the seat. Both methods help to calm. If the child feels sick, put 2 drops of the 'Motion sickness mix' (above) on a tissue, for him or her to sniff.

Essential oils that help

ginger
rosemary
peppermint
coriander
eucalyptus radiata
cardamom

PREVENTION

 Have the child lie down with his or her eyes closed on the back seat of the car. Ensure the seatbelt is used. If this is difficult, have the child lay back in the seat with cushions supporting the head.

 Some children find it easier if they always look directly ahead during car travel.

 It sometimes helps if the child can nibble on dry biscuits, or sip water/tea while travelling.

 Open the window to get fresh air; or, if in a traffic jam, close any windows in order to keep pollution out of the vehicle.

 Don't make an issue of motion sickness before travel as this may upset the child and precondition him or her to be sick for real.

Mumps

Mumps is caused by an airborne virus, which affects the parotid salivary glands. The most characteristic symptom of mumps is large swellings just below the ears. It's usually caught in the same way as so many other conditions – by people sneezing or coughing infected droplets into the air – although other direct contact with an infected person's saliva will also transmit the virus. The symptoms appear a couple of weeks after infection, and last for a few days. The virus is contagious during the two days before the glands swell, and for around 10 days afterwards.

Usually mumps is fairly harmless, but there can be serious complications. In rare cases, the brain can become affected and meningitis may develop. Occasionally, permanent deafness results from mumps. Sometimes other glands become involved, particularly the testes, ovaries and pancreas. Watch to make sure your son's testicles don't become swollen – if they do, inform your doctor straight away. If a boy catches mumps during puberty, it can result in sterility. The same is the case for adult men who did not contract mumps as a child.

Signs and symptoms

 large swellings on one or both sides of the neck (the glands), just below the ears; can be very sore

 difficulty in swallowing; dry mouth

 mild fever

 headache; earache

 sometimes swollen face and tongue

 in serious cases – painful, swollen testicles (boys); lower abdominal ovarian pain (girls)

Method

Baths

First, mix the following essential oils:

lavender – 4 drops
geranium – 4 drops

mandarin – 4 drops.

Dilute 4 drops of the mix in 1 teaspoon vegetable oil, and add to the bath

water. The amount above is enough essential oil for three baths.

Compresses

Essential oils can be used in compresses applied over the swollen glands. Some children prefer warm compresses, while others prefer the water to be cool – older children can be asked which feels best to them. To $\frac{1}{2}$ pint water, add 4 drops of the following mix:

eucalyptus radiata – 10 drops
thyme linalol – 5 drops
lavender 4 drops.

Put the compress in the water, squeeze it out, and apply to both glands in the neck, under the ears.

Back and neck oil

First, make a mix of essential oils using the following:

lavender – 15 drops
chamomile roman – 5 drops
chamomile german – 5 drops
eucalyptus radiata – 5 drops.

Dilute the essential oil mix in 1 teaspoon vegetable oil, using the following amount according to the age of the child:

under 5 years – 3 drops
6–8 years – 4 drops
over 9 years – 5 drops.

Use the diluted oil to massage the back. Also apply to the neck – but without massaging.

Do this twice a day.

Mumps mix

The following mix can be used in the two methods outlined below. Follow directions for each method. First, mix the following essential oils together:

thyme linalol – 5 drops
lavender – 5 drops
ravensara – 10 drops.

Over 7s
Only use this method if your child is over 7 years of age.

Apply 1 drop of the 'Mumps mix' above directly on the swollen gland under the ears. If both sides are swollen, use 1 drop on each side.

Use this method no more than once a day (bedtime is best).

Abdominal rub
Dilute 3 drops of the 'Mumps mix' above in 1 teaspoon vegetable oil.

Smooth over the lower abdomen, avoiding the genital area.

Do not use on the testicles.

Essential oils that help

tea tree
coriander
lemon
lavender
chamomile roman
ravensara
niaouli
helichrysum
eucalyptus radiata

Other care

Give your child plenty of fluid, avoiding citrus fruit juices and other acidic drinks. It can be difficult to swallow easily at this time, so give your child soups and mashed-up or liquidized foods. Ice cream will help to cool the throat.

Some children get relief by having something warm against their neck, such as a warm towel, warm pack or hot-water bottle – but make sure it is warm, not hot. Other children prefer something cool against the neck, such as a cool compress. Ask your child what feels best.

When to get help

Contact your doctor as soon as you suspect mumps. Call your doctor again if (in the case of a boy) the testicles become swollen or (in the case of a girl) she experiences lower abdominal pain. Your doctor should also be told if your child's neck gets stiff and painful; if there are headaches; or if the condition does not improve within 10 days.

PREVENTION

 It is possible to be inoculated against mumps. The vaccines are cultured on egg protein, so if your child is allergic to eggs discuss that with your doctor before proceeding.

Muscles – overexercised

See also Strains – ligaments.

Children are supposed to be active, but sometimes they overdo it – playing sports, running, cycling, doing gymnastics, exercises, too many dance lessons, or just climbing and jumping all day. Overexercised muscles are sometimes the result.

Signs and symptoms

 aching muscles, sometimes with pain

 usually occurs in the legs and arms

 pain worse in the morning

Method

When a child has overdone the exercise, or been playing too zealously, the best course of action is to apply a body oil and rub it into the muscles, just before your child has a warm bath. This helps the essential oils sink into the skin so they can warm and soothe the muscles. The child should soak in the bath for a while to give the muscles a chance to relax, so give older children a book to read, and younger children a toy to play with. This relaxing routine may give children an appreciation of relaxing baths, which in later life could provide them with an escape from the stresses of life.

The following massage oil and bath method is not to be used just because your child has been physically active, but because after the activity they complain of muscle ache, and are in need of care.

Essential oils that help

ginger
chamomile roman
marjoram
cardamom
rosemary
helichrysum

Overexercised muscles, pre-bath oil mix

The following routine will reduce the likelihood of sore, stiff muscles in the morning.

It is most effective if carried out just before bedtime.

First, mix the following essential oils together:

marjoram – 3 drops
chamomile roman – 2 drops
lavender – 2 drops
ginger – 2 drops.

See page 27 for the number of drops of essential oils to dilute in 1 teaspoon vegetable oil, depending on the age of your child.

Apply enough of the oil to cover the skin, over the aching or sore muscles, and rub in.

Then let your child have a warm bath, where they should soak and relax.

If your child is very dirty, after a football game for example, he or she should have a shower before the muscle oil is applied and the child gets in the bath.

If stiffness continues in the morning, massage a small amount of the diluted mix into the affected area, and repeat the bath.

Other care

It's important that, in the case of overexercised muscles, only warmth is applied, because it increases the flow of blood to the area. Put a hot-water bottle or heat bag against the overexercised muscle or, if the affected muscle is in the leg or arm, wrap it in warm towels.

When to get help

Get help if the pain is very severe, and if the child can't walk with ease or freely lift the affected limb.

PREVENTION

 Teach your child to stretch and do warm-up exercises before – and after – doing any sports, dance or other strenuous physical activity.

Nappy rash

This is a common complaint that can affect all babies, but especially those with sensitive skin, prone to allergies, infantile eczema or psoriasis. The baby might be allergic to certain chemical baby wipes, cleaning materials, detergents and soaps. Babies who have candida (sometimes induced by antibiotics) can also develop a rash.

Nappy rash is most commonly caused by wearing wet or soiled nappies for long periods of time. Faeces can break down the urine components and release ammonia into the area.

If not treated, nappy rash can become severe and infected with bacteria or fungi. If this happens, the rash will have small, blister-like raised areas or small, pus-infected spots. Action must be taken immediately to stop the spread of infection.

At all times, avoid putting harsh, dry material in contact with the area, because this causes more discomfort.

Signs and symptoms

 affects buttocks, creases of the leg, groin area, genitals

 redness of skin, inflammation, rashes of various types, scaly patches, or rough skin

Method

Prior to treatment

Rinse off urine and/or faeces as soon as possible with mild soap and water. Use cotton wool, making sure none is left on the skin. Pat the area dry using a clean, soft natural material, such as muslin or cheesecloth.

After washing

Add a true herbal hydrolat of chamomile roman or lavender to the final rinse water.

If not available, make your own 'water'. Follow the directions on page 18, using, in 1 pint water:

chamomile german –
4 drops
lavender 4 drops.

Nappy rash oil

Heat up 75 ml (3 ounces) organic jojoba oil and 30 ml (1 ounce) organic olive oil. Leave to get cold.

Meantime, mix:

chamomile german –
8 drops
lavender – 4 drops
ravensara – 4 drops.

(If candida is the cause, add 8 drops of tea tree oil to the mix.)

Now mix the essential oils into the cold vegetable oils. Apply a small amount at each nappy change until the rash goes. Try to avoid the penis, testicle or vulval area.

Do not use over cuts or cracks in the skin.

Baths

Mix (in 1 tablespoon full-fat milk):

chamomile german –
1 drop
lavender – 1 drop.

Then add to the surface of the bath water and swish around well. Avoid getting the oil on baby's face during the bath.

Essential oils that help

In general	With infected pustules	With candida albicans
chamomile german	lavender	geranium
chamomile roman	ravensara	manuka
lavender	thyme linalol	tea tree
palmarosa	tea tree	thyme linalol
yarrow		

Other care

In general

1 or 2 drops of chamomile german can be added to each tablespoon of zinc oxide cream.

With infected pustules (spots)

Colloidal silver solution can be combined with essential oils.

With candida albicans

Natural (non-flavoured), bio-active yoghurt can be combined with tea tree and manuka essential oils and applied over the affected area of skin.

When to get help

If pus can be seen in small spots, or there are blister-like areas, see a doctor before treating with anything, or if the condition does not improve within four days.

PREVENTION

   Combine 120 ml (4 ounces) organic almond oil and 30 ml (1 ounce) organic olive oil, and gently apply a tiny amount after each nappy change.

   Or apply another water-repellent oil or cream.

✿ It is important to get air to the area at least once a day. Leave the nappy off for a time, when practical to do so.

✿ Change nappies frequently.

✿ Keep the skin dry (apart from the oils or creams as mentioned above).

Pneumonia

Pneumonia attacks the lungs, and the infection can be caused by a virus, bacteria or fungus. There are two types: one affects the air passages and then spreads to the lungs; the other affects the lobes of the lungs. One or both lungs can be infected.

Pneumonia can be caught by breathing in infected air. It can also develop from bacteria that are normally present in the nose and throat of the infected person, especially when their resistance to disease is generally low. As the symptoms are so like those of many other diseases, it can be difficult for a parent to decide if the child has the infection or not. It can start with cold-like symptoms, often with a cough. The treatment of pneumonia with pharmacological antibiotics has been very good.

Signs and symptoms

✿ can start with cold-like symptoms: cough; stuffed-up nose; tiredness

✿ high temperature or fever, yet the child may feel chilly

✿ difficulty in breathing; may wheeze

✿ chest pains; lung ache or pain

✿ child produces phlegm

headache

 abdominal pains

 lips and nails look bluish

Method

Pneumonia mix

The following mix can be used in several ways. Follow the directions in the boxes below. First, mix the following:

ravensara – 10 drops
eucalyptus citriodora – 10 drops
niaouli – 10 drops
thyme linalol – 5 drops.

Body rub
A massage over the back and upper chest can make breathing easier.

Use a small amount of the following mix each time:

15 ml ($^1/2$ ounce) vegetable oil
pneumonia mix above – 10 drops.

Baths
Dilute 3 drops of the pneumonia mix above in $^1/2$ teaspoon vegetable oil.

If your child is over 7, use all the mix. If your child is 6 or under, use half the amount.

Add to the bath water, and swish around well before your child gets in.

Diffuser
In one of the room methods, use:

pneumonia mix (see above) – 5 drops
cinnamon – 5 drops.

If you use a diffuser, do not leave it in your child's room overnight.

Tissue or pillow
Put 1–2 drops of the pneumonia mix on a tissue, for your child to sniff when needed.

Put 1–2 drops of the pneumonia mix on pillows – under the corner, and away from the eyes.

223

Fevers

If your child has a fever, try one of the remedies below to bring the temperature down.

Sponge method
This method is particularly helpful if your child is hot and sticky.

Prepare a bowl of lukewarm – not cold – water, to which you've added 2 drops of lavender. Soak a sponge, squeeze it out, and use to wipe down your child's body.

Vinegar method
This method has been a favourite with Europeans for generations.

Follow the instructions for the vinegar method given under Fever (page 144).

Compress and massage
Sleep is important. For a method that will both help to bring down the fever and help your child to sleep, follow the compress and massage instructions given under Fever (page 144).

Essential oils that help

ravensara
tea tree
niaouli
thyme linalol
elemi

Other care

Give your child plenty of liquids and get him or her to rest. If you prop the child up in bed, this will ease the coughing and make breathing easier. Open the windows so air can circulate freely.

Bedsocks

Put the following essential oils on the inside sole of two bedsocks:

thyme linalol – I drop
ginger – I drop.

Put the socks on your child's feet, and keep the feet warm.

When to get help

Contact your doctor immediately if your child has any of the symptoms listed above and you think he or she may have contracted pneumonia. Once diagnosed, get additional medical help as soon as possible if your child experiences any difficulty in breathing.

PREVENTION

Prevention is directed at trying to ensure other members of the family do not contract pneumonia. Elderly people and babies are especially at risk.

   Keep other members of the household away from the child with pneumonia.

   Other members of the household could use 4 drops of the pneumonia mix of essential oils in the bath.

   Diffuse anti-viral essential oils throughout the home.

Psoriasis

Psoriasis is a skin condition with dry, scaly patches, and can come on in childhood or adulthood. The severity of the condition changes very much from person to person: there may be small patches that come up all over the body; or larger patches, on the elbows and knees, for example. In really severe cases, a large part of the body's surface can be covered. There are different types of the condition – in children the most common type is a mild form called glutate psoriasis.

Why a person should develop psoriasis is unknown, but various triggers can cause outbreaks, including having an infection, an injury on the skin, or being under stress. The winter months can make it worse because the skin isn't being exposed to the sun. Psoriasis appears to run in families, and you often find that other members of the child's family have hayfever or are asthmatic.

aromatherapy for your child

Signs and symptoms

 can start with tiny bumps of reddish-pink flaky skin areas – behind the knees, in the crook of the elbow, lower back, on the scalp or hairline

 scales look quite silvery and flake off easily

 skin may crack and become painful, therefore risk of infection

 joints can swell, ache or become painful

Method

Oat baths

Oat baths can be wonderfully soothing to the skin. Use raw organic oats or oatmeal. Put a pile of oats or oatmeal on to a piece of material, and add the essential oils to them. Securely tie the bundle and attach it to the bath tap, so the water runs through the oats before reaching the bath. There are four baths to choose from – different children respond differently to particular oils.

To bath 1, add:

chamomile german – 4 drops.

To bath 2, add:

bergamot – 4 drops.

To bath 3, add:

spikenard – 1 drop.

To bath 4, add:

lavender – 2 drops.

Oil bath

Use half of this mix in a bath:

1 teaspoon almond oil
lavender – 1 drop
bergamot – 1 drop
geranium – 1 drop
chamomile roman – 1 drop.

Swish the water around well before your child gets in the bath.

All types of psoriasis are different, and a lot depends on the constitution of the child. There is no overall remedy that will be effective for all children.

Bicarb bath

First, add the following essential oils to 100g bicarbonate of soda:

lavender – 2 drops
chamomile german – 1 drop.

Mix in well with a spoon, then add to the bath water. Swish the water around well before your child gets in.

Skin oil 1

Smooth a small amount over the patches of dry, flaky skin. Mix together well:

30 ml (1 ounce) sesame seed oil
30 ml (1 ounce) pure virgin olive oil.

Then add:

red carrot oil – 25 drops
borage seed oil – 5 drops
geranium – 3 drops

Mix together well.

Skin oil 2

Smooth a small amount over the patches of dry, flaky skin. Mix together well:

30 ml (1 ounce) calendula-infused oil
bergamot – 4 drops
chamomile roman – 3 drops.

Essential oils that help

chamomile german
chamomile roman
lavender
bergamot
spikenard
rose otto

Other care

Certain foods make the condition worse – dairy products, wheat products, additives, preservatives, food colouring, and manufactured foods. Fizzy drinks, condiments, prepackaged sauces and other preprepared foods are all likely to make the condition worse.

It may seem like a daunting task, but the long-term future of your child's psoriasis may depend to some degree on totally adjusting their diet, and possibly that of the family as well. You may like to follow the Cave Man Eating Plan given on page 24. Basically, if a food walked, swam or flew, you can eat it. If it grows out of the ground, that's fine, and if it's raw, that's even better. Cereals, flours and condiments should all be organic. The whole family will enjoy more home cooking, and will feel better for it. Cutting out certain additives may even improve your child's behaviour. Buying organic can cost more, but you save on drinks and preprepared foods – and you may actually end up getting more for your money. It's got to be worth trying for a month.

When to get help

If you suspect your child may be developing psoriasis, consult your doctor. The general prescription is hydrocortisone and, if it becomes more of a problem, steroid creams. Tar creams or baths may also be recommended. In European hospitals, a popular treatment for severe cases is the ultraviolet light from sunbeds.

Rashes

See also Rashes – newborn.

Skin rashes are caused by many things and are often a symptom of infection or disease. They may be a reaction of the body's immune system as it tries to fight off an invader. Rashes are also allergic reactions to something in the atmosphere already; something that has touched or bitten the skin; or something that has been eaten. Parasites can sometimes cause rashes, which can also result from a serious blood condition. There are so many possible causes of skin rash that it is often hard to identify the cause in every case.

If there is a rash on your child's body, you need to look for other symptoms or causes. Has the child got a temperature or fever, or other signs of illness? Has your child been playing in long grass or near woods? Is the rash spreading? If so, note this down. Blood poisoning – septicaemia – causes a rash that does not fade temporarily when a clear glass is pressed against it (see *Meningitis*). This rash starts as a group of very tiny blood spots, but these rapidly get bigger, when they resemble fresh bruises with bleeding under the skin. If your child's rash matches this description, do not wait for medical help – take him or her immediately to the nearest medical facility and insist on being seen instantly.

Signs and symptoms

Rashes come in all shapes and sizes, and anywhere on the body. Some may be raised or bumpy, while others are flat. Some are more like blisters; with others, the surrounding tissue may be swollen. The rash might be pink, red or purple. The rash might be a series of spots joined together or a continuous area of similarly disturbed skin. Some rashes are distinctive, and indicate a particular cause, while others could be caused by a variety of things. To help you identify the cause of your child's rash, refer to the 'Signs and symptoms' lists in the individual sections. These are some of the causes of rashes:

 Virus chickenpox; rubella (German measles); slapped-cheek disease; hand, foot and mouth disease

 Bacteria meningitis; impetigo; scarlet fever

 Fungus ringworm; thrush

 Parasite scabies

 Allergic reaction hives; contact dermatitis

 Allergic reaction poison ivy; poison oak; poison sumbac; other plants; chemicals; medication; foods (e.g. strawberries, cherries and eggs)

 Insect bite bees, wasps, fleas, ants, mosquitoes

Possible causes for newborns are thema toxicum, cradle cap, prickly heat (see *Rashes – newborn*)

Method

Baths

If your child has a rash, keep the skin cool and give your child soothing baths.

Add the following to a bath of tepid to warm water:

1 tablespoon bicarbonate of soda
1 tablespoon baking soda
chamomile german – 2 drops
lavender – 2 drops.

Essential oils that help

chamomile german
lavender
chamomile roman
helichrysum
niaouli
eucalyptus radiata

Other care

Try to stop your child from scratching the rash, as this might lead to infection.

When to get help

Get medical help if your child has a temperature or fever. Also seek medical attention if the rash gets worse and spreads; if the rash is infected with pus or is bleeding; or if it does not improve after 48 hours.

Rashes – newborn

Some figures say that 50 per cent of newborn babies have rashes – certainly it is very common. The cause is not really known, but a rash could just be the baby's skin getting acclimatized to the outside world after spending nine months in the womb; or a reaction to the air on the skin or to wearing clothing. It's always worrying when a newborn has a rash, especially for a first-time parent, so do get reassurance from your doctor.

Signs and symptoms

 slightly raised red rash, on any part of the body

 sometimes with a few pimples

 lasts 7–14 days

Method

I prefer not to use essential oils on these sort of newborn babies' rashes unless it is causing distress. If your baby's skin is very dry, use a small amount of pure, virgin, organic olive oil and smooth it on to your baby's skin. Try to avoid baby oils, creams and lotions, many of which contain mineral products. The following two methods can safely be used on newborns if you follow the directions exactly. In warm weather, try to leave baby's skin exposed to the air as much as possible, rather than covering it in wool or other warm clothing.

Body oil

This oil is effective in clearing up a newborn skin rash. Very little essential oil is used in the following mix, and you will only need to use a tiny amount each time.

First, mix the following:

30 ml (1 ounce) virgin, organic olive oil
chamomile german – 1 drop.

Put a tiny amount of the oil in the palm of one hand and rub both hands together. This spreads the oil so you don't use too much, and helps to make the oil warm and comfortable to the baby. Then smooth your hands over the affected areas of baby's skin.

Do not leave baby's skin greasy – dab any excess off with a soft piece of material.

Hydrolat/water lotion

See page 18 for how to make an essential oil 'water'.

First, combine the following:

8 ml ($^1/_4$ ounce) lavender hydrolat (or 'water')
8 ml ($^1/_4$ ounce) chamomile (or 'water').

Take half this amount, and add to 8 ml ($^1/_4$ ounce) warm – not hot – pure bottled water.

Add a few grains of salt.

Use a small sponge to dab gently on baby's rash, then pat dry.

Essential oil that helps

chamomile german

When to get help

Consult your doctor if you are unsure what the rash is, or if it doesn't clear up in 14 days. If any children in the home or neighbourhood have a contagious infection of any kind, get medical advice.

Ringworm

Strictly speaking, ringworm refers to a large group of different fungal infections. What people generally know as ringworm is a skin infection that looks a bit like a bull's eye, circular or ring-shaped, with an unaffected area in the middle. The outer ring of ringworm marks the active area of the fungus. The centre heals as the fungus moves outwards, making the circle larger.

Ringworm is caused by a highly contagious fungus called *tinea*, and can spread quickly around a school. It's caught by contact with the fungus, either directly by touching infected skin, or indirectly by sharing the belongings of an infected person, such as clothes, hats, brushes, combs, towels, facecloths or pillows. It's most common in children between the ages of 2 and 10, and can last up to six weeks.

Signs and symptoms

    reddish-pink, circular, slightly raised mark on the skin – the centre is unaffected

    found anywhere on the body, but particularly: the face, limbs, groin and scalp – where it can cause patches of hair loss

    patches can enlarge; the area can become itchy with scaly skin

    sometimes pus-filled, lumpy swellings

    due to the child scratching the ringworm, fingernails may be infected – pitted, thick and discoloured

Method

Scalp treatment

First, mix the following essential oils:

manuka – 10 drops
neem – 20 drops
tea tree – 20 drops
palmarosa – 10 drops
geranium – 10 drops.

Put 20 drops of the above mix in 120 ml (4 ounces) plain, anti-allergen, mild, baby shampoo and mix well. Use enough to shampoo the hair, and rinse well with water.

Then, dilute 4 drops of the essential oil mix above in 1 tablespoon sesame oil, and apply enough to cover the scalp – make sure none reaches the eyes, ears, nose or mouth.

Leave it in place for 10 minutes. Then wash the hair again, using plain shampoo.

As a final rinse water, use 60 ml (2 ounces) water to which you have added 3 drops of the essential oil mix above. Pour it over the scalp and hair, making sure to avoid the eyes, ears, nose and mouth.

Treat all the family with the same method, whether they're infected or not.

Shower method

A warm shower will help to ease the itchy skin. Directly after the shower, while your child is still standing in the shower cubicle, gently pour chamomile hydrolat/'water' over your child's body (see page 18 for how to prepare essential oil hydrolats or 'waters').

Ringworm mix

This can be used in the two methods below. Follow the instructions below.

First, mix the following essential oils:

tea tree – 5 drops
manuka – 5 drops
neem – 8 drops.

Neat
Use 1 drop of the ringworm mix above, directly over the infected area.

Do this three times a day.

Evening body oil
Dilute 3 drops of the ringworm mix above in 1 teaspoon sesame oil.

In the evening, use to rub over the whole body, avoiding the genital area. If the ringworm is very itchy, use over the affected area during the day as well.

Essential oils that help

lavender
tea tree
manuka
neem
palmarosa
geranium

When to get help

Get medical advice if you are not sure that your child's skin condition is ringworm. Also get help if the ringworm is on the face or scalp, if it seems to be infected, or if it doesn't clear up after two weeks of any form of treatment.

PREVENTION

Prevention consists of trying to stop the spread of infection.

   Cover the area with a dressing.

   Make sure the affected child's facecloth, towel, pillows and clothes are not shared.

   Until the infection has cleared up, try to stop the affected child having close contact with other children and family members.

Rubella (German measles)

Rubella is a milder form of measles. It's inconvenient, but not harmful – unless it's caught by a woman during the first four months of pregnancy, when it can cause serious defects in the unborn child. If a girl child has not had German measles in her childhood, she can be vaccinated against it when she's a young woman, so that if she comes into contact with rubella when she's pregnant later it doesn't cause her problems. The most important thing if your child has rubella is to keep him or her out of contact with pregnant women until the infection has passed.

Rubella is a viral infection that causes a rash – which may start with just a small patch, usually behind the ears, but can spread and cover almost the whole body. It lasts anything from 3 – 15 days. Other symptoms may include mild fever and swollen glands. It's sometimes difficult to tell from the symptoms whether a child has rubella or another type of rash or infection.

Rubella is an airborne infection, which seems to be most active during the spring months. It's spread by an infected person sneezing or coughing, and the infected air being breathed in. The incubation time is generally 14–21 days, although the rash can appear as early as three days after the virus has been contracted. A child is infectious during the time they have the rash and for up to seven days after it has disappeared. Most children are immunized against this disease, but some still contract rubella even after immunization.

Signs and symptoms

 runny nose; other cold-like symptoms

 small rash appears – usually starts behind the ears, then spreads to the body

 sometimes – mild fever; glands behind the ears are swollen

Method

Aloe vera bath

Use 4 drops of the essential oil mix below, added to 30 ml (1 ounce) aloe vera water and 30 ml (1 ounce) lavender water. Add the entire mix to the bath water:

lavender – 5 drops
chamomile roman – 3 drops
chamomile german – 3 drops
bergamot – 4 drops.

Use 4 drops only. Swish the water around well before the child gets in the bath.

Bath to help sleep

The following combination of essential oils will not only soothe the rash, but help the child get a good night's sleep. Put the following essential oils in 1 teaspoon vegetable oil, then add to the bath water (swish around well before the child gets in):

geranium – 2 drops
lavender – 2 drops
petitgrain – 1 drop.

Swollen glands oil

Use a blob of oil about the size of a five-pence piece. Apply gently over the glands behind both ears, and down the neck and into the armpits.

1 teaspoon vegetable oil
thyme linalol – 5 drops.

When a child has rubella, rest and plenty of fluid are the order of the day. Use an anti-viral mix of essential oil in the diffuser or spray methods to help stop the spread of the virus to other members of the household. The spots in the rash can be very itchy, and soothing baths help stop the irritation. Use warm, not hot, water in baths.

Essential oils that help

lavender
thyme linalol
chamomile roman
tea tree
geranium
bergamot
ravensara

Other care

Keep your child away from pregnant women, and other members of the family. Put your child to bed only if they are feeling unwell.

When to get help

Always inform your doctor if your child catches rubella. If your child complains of a stiff neck, or if his or her temperature rises, consult your doctor again.

PREVENTION

 Immunization is available.

 To help prevent the infection spreading to other people, use anti-viral essential oils around the home – in the diffuser and spray methods.

Shock

Shock often follows after an injury, blood loss, pain, fear, bereavement or an emotional trauma such as seeing an accident or violent incident. The shock can come on immediately or very slowly. Shock is very dangerous and can cause physical damage if not treated medically. There are many circumstances in which shock may occur, and whenever there has been physical damage to the child, or another person within their sight, or emotional trauma, the symptoms should be looked for, bearing in mind that the shock may occur some time after the shocking event.

Signs and symptoms

 child feels cold

 clammy skin

 blood appears to drain from the face, which is very pale

 dry mouth

 breathing quickens and/or becomes shallow; hyperventilation

 pulse can quicken and/or become faint

 child is unable to move – frozen and trance-like

 child carries on, but with slow, mechanical movements, little reaction, and staring eyes

Method

Inhalation

Since mankind first noticed the power of smell, essential oils and other fragrant materials have been given to people in shock to smell. 'Smelling salts' are not appropriate in cases of shock.

Use 1 drop of any of the following essential oils. Put the essential oil on to a tissue or piece of cloth and pass it under the child's nose. In an emergency, just pass the bottle itself under the child's nose.

chamomile roman
geranium
lemon.

Comforting hand or foot massage

A child often needs comforting after having mild shock which requires no medication or hospital treatment. This may be the case if the child has had a scary experience.

A light, comforting massage of the hands or feet (or both) can work wonders, especially when combined with cuddles.

Use the following mix:

1 teaspoon vegetable oil
mandarin (or tangerine) – 1 drop
petitgrain – 1 drop.

Essential oils that help

lemon
geranium
chamomile roman
rose

Other care

If an injury has occurred, do not move your child. If there is no neck, back or head injury, raise the head slightly, but not the legs. If the child has not been injured at all, lie him or her down, and raise the legs above head level, to encourage the flow of blood to the heart and brain. To keep the child warm, cover up with whatever is available.

There are certain preprepared natural remedies for shock – Dr Bach's Rescue Remedy or Five Flower Essence Healing Herbs; homoeopathic arnica tablets; Front Line Mother Essences.

When to get help

If your child is in shock, he or she needs immediate emergency medical attention.

PREVENTION

If a disaster has occurred:

 Cover your child.

 Comfort your child by rubbing his or her hands.

Sinusitis

Sinusitis is an inflammation of the lining of the sinuses. There are many causes, including hayfever, allergy, nasal injury, being in a smoky atmosphere, ear problems, or infections of the throat, teeth, gums, colds and flu.

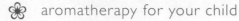

Signs and symptoms

 nasal congestion

 headache

 sore and swollen eyes; can feel as if they are throbbing

 pain around the cheek bones and forehead

 fatigue; feeling generally unwell

 in serious cases – a thick, yellowy-green nasal discharge

Method

Compresses

Compresses can help relieve the congestion. You can use either warm or hot compresses, depending on which your child finds more effective at the time.

First, add the following essential oils to a bowl containing 1 pint warm or hot water:

rosemary – 4 drops

eucalyptus radiata – 2 drops
ravensara – 6 drops.

Place a compress or facecloth in the water, squeeze it out well and place over your child's forehead. Make sure no water goes into the eyes. An older child can hold the compress in place. As the compress starts to dry, have another ready to use. You should get at least four compresses out of one bowl of water.

Steam methods

Steam often helps the child to breathe more easily, and essential oils can be added in the following methods.

Bowl method
Put a bowl of steaming water in your child's room, and add the following essential oils:

ravensara – 4 drops
niaouli – 4 drops
chamomile roman – 4 drops.

Make sure the bowl is out of reach of children and pets.

Inhalation
An older child can use the inhalation method. Make up the mix of essential oils given under 'Bowl method', and use 4 drops in a bowl of steaming water.

Your child should inhale this, leaning over the bowl with his or her head covered, and mouth and eyes closed.

Menthol crystals (available from chemists) can also be used in this inhalation.

Bathrooms
If the sinuses are really bad and your child can find no relief, the very steamy atmosphere of a bathroom may help.

Run a very hot bath, and keep the door closed. Have your child sit in the bathroom – but not in the bath itself – and inhale the steam through the nose.

Add the complete sinusitis mix (see below) to the water – this is a lot of drops, but remember that nobody is actually getting in the bath.

Sinusitis mix

The following mix of essential oils can be used in the methods below. Follow the instructions in each box.

First, mix the following essential oils together:

ravensara – 6 drops
niaouli – 5 drops
eucalyptus radiata – 2 drops
chamomile roman – 4 drops.

Forehead oil
Put a tiny amount of the following mix on one fingertip and smooth it over the forehead and nose, being careful to avoid the eye area:

1 teaspoon vegetable oil
sinusitis mix (above) – 3 drops
chamomile german – 1 drop.

With a tissue, gently dab off any excess oil that has not soaked into the skin.

Tissue method
Put 1 drop of the 'Sinusitis mix' on a tissue. Give it to your child to inhale during the day.

Pillow method
At night, put 1 drop of the 'Sinusitis mix' on your child's pillow – under a corner and away from the eyes. Use extra pillows to prop your child up higher.

Essential oils that help

ravensara
niaouli
tea tree
chamomile roman
eucalyptus radiata
rosemary

Other care

Salt-water nose drops are often used, and are available at chemists. A hot, dry, stuffy atmosphere makes the condition worse, so keep your child's room aired, and use a humidifier or similar method to keep the air moist overnight. Give your child plenty of fluids to drink, including fruit juices, and avoid dairy products for a while as these can cause more mucus in the body.

When to get help

Get medical help if the headache turns into a throb, if the condition lasts for longer than three days, or if there is a thick yellowy-green nasal discharge that lasts longer than three days.

Slapped-cheek disease (Erythema infectiosum)

Slapped-cheek disease is a contagious rash caused by a virus – Human Parovirus B19. The rash generally lasts no longer than 24 days, although in some children it will fade and then reappear. The virus is not harmful to most children, but it can have a bad effect on children with a blood disorder, lowered immunity condition or cancer. Pregnant women, too, should try to avoid it, as it can cause anaemia or miscarriage

Slapped-cheek disease is very common among children of primary school age, especially during the winter and spring months. It's caught simply by breathing in affected air. Because it's very contagious during the two weeks before the rash appears, it's difficult to control. Once the rash has appeared, the child is no longer contagious, but by then the virus could have passed halfway through a school. In warmer climates especially, the rash can appear and then disappear, then appear again, and so on for weeks. This can make it difficult to know for sure whether the child is contagious or not.

Things are further complicated by the fact that there are often no obvious symptoms to slapped-cheek disease disease at all – the child just feels generally unwell, with aches and pains and irritability. The child might have a slight fever, and less energy – and may just want to lie around all day. Slapped-cheek disease can even be mistaken for the common cold.

Signs and symptoms

 a rash on the cheeks

 in some children, rash may spread to other parts of the body, such as the legs and arms

 older children – often no rash, but instead aches and pains in their joints

Method

Especially if you have other children in the household, or a pregnant woman, spray the air with anti-viral essential oils (see 'Anti-infectious air spray' on page 45). Baths can help soothe the skin if your child has the rash (there are several sorts to choose from). Aside from those below, you could try one of the baths outlined in the *Chickenpox* or *Eczema* sections (see pages 97 and 138).

Oat bath

Here is an oat bath that can be prepared quickly. Add the following to the bath water and swish around well before the child gets in:

1 large tablespoon oatmeal
1 handful sea salt
lavender – 1 drop
chamomile german – 1 drop
tea tree – 1 drop.

Soothing bath

First, add these essential oils to a cup of bicarbonate of soda:

lavender – 2 drops
chamomile german – 1 drop
helichrysum – 1 drop.

Then mix in well with a spoon before adding to the bath water.

Adolescent joint rub

If your child is an adolescent with joint pains caused by slapped-cheek disease, mix the following together and rub a small amount over all the joints just before the child has a warm bath:

60 ml (2 ounces) vegetable oil
rosemary – 5 drops
lavender – 7 drops
marjoram – 8 drops
thyme linalol – 5 drops.

Essential oils that help

lavender
lemon
chamomile roman
thyme linalol
chamomile german
helichrysum
geranium
cardamom

Other care

Spray the air with anti-viral essential oils (see 'Anti-infectious air spray' on page 45).

When to get help

Get medical attention if your child also has a blood disorder, or a condition with lowered immunity, or cancer.

PREVENTION

   If a child in the home has slapped-cheek disease, keep them away from other children.

   Spray the air with anti-viral essential oils (see 'Anti-infectious air spray' on page 45).

Sore throat ('strep throat')

Children often complain of sore throats, which more often than not have gone by the next morning. This sort of throat irritation is usually caused by a bacteria or virus. 'Strep' throat is caused by the *Streptococcus* bacteria, and usually clears up within a few days. However, a sore throat can be a symptom of a more serious condition, and certain steps need to be taken to decide if this is the case.

Take your child's temperature, and check whether his or her glands are swollen. Ask if there is difficulty in swallowing. Use a spoon to hold down your child's tongue, and check to see if the throat or tonsils have any inflammation, redness or swelling. Look to see if there are any white spots. A sore throat could be a symptom of several conditions, including a cold, flu, laryngitis, mumps, nephritis, rheumatic fever, scarlet fever and tonsillitis.

Signs and symptoms

   pain in the throat; difficulty in swallowing

   swollen lymph glands

   red and swollen tonsils

   white spots on the tonsils

Method

Sore throat drink

Drinks can help ease the soreness in the throat. The following soothing drink can be given to children over the age of 2. If your child is younger, omit the lemon essential oil. First, mix together well:

240 ml (8 ounces) hot water
1 teaspoon runny honey
2 tablespoons cooking rose-water
juice of 1 lemon
lemon essential oil – 1 drop.

Then pour the mixture through an unbleached paper coffee-filter.

When the drink is cool, give it to your child to sip. Cover the drink, and leave it by your child's side, so he or she can sip it when there is a need to do so. Very young children can be given the drink by spoon.

Throat oil

Use a small amount of the following oil to rub over the throat area.

First, mix together the following essential oils:

tea tree – 4 drops
lemon – 2 drops

ravensara – 5 drops
thyme linalol – 4 drops
manuka (or additional tea tree) – 5 drops.

Dilute 5 drops of the mix in 1 teaspoon vegetable oil. This will be enough for several applications.

Swollen glands oil

Thyme linalol or manuka essential oil can be used in high dosage over the glands on either side of the neck.

Put I drop of your chosen essential oil on a fingertip, plus I drop of vegetable oil. Rub your fingertips together, and smooth over the glands.

Essential oils that help

tea tree
chamomile roman
thyme linalol
ravensara
helichrysum
manuka
ginger
eucalyptus radiata
cajuput
geranium

Other care

See the advice in *Laryngitis*. Keep your child away from school, give them plenty to drink and liquidize all foods. To soothe the throat, give your child ice cream and frozen fruit-juice lollies. If the throat is inflamed, warm compresses applied to the throat sometimes help.

When to get help

Consult your doctor if there are white spots anywhere in the mouth or throat, if your child has a temperature or fever, a rash, headache, or aches and pains.

Splinters

A splinter is a small foreign object embedded in the skin or flesh. Most splinters a child is likely to get will be from wood, thorns or plastic – rarely is metal involved, unless your child spends time in garages or workshops where metal shavings are present. Most splinters can easily be removed at home.

Signs and symptoms

 small object is visible beneath the skin

 pain; soreness

 if not removed, can become infected

Method

If the splinter is visible and can be firmly grasped, remove it very carefully with a pair of tweezers. The whole splinter must be removed to avoid the risk of infection. If the splinter is caught in the skin, it may help to soften the area with warm water before trying to remove the splinter. But don't try this if the splinter is made of wood, as soaking will just make the wood soft and therefore more likely to break, and it will become impossible to remove it easily. After removing the splinter, wash the area well with soap and water, and apply 1 drop of one of the following essential oils.

Essential oils that help

myrrh
thyme linalol
tea tree
manuka

Other care

Use disinfectant or tea tree in the washing water. If the hole in the skin is large enough to require covering with a sticking plaster, keep an eye on it to make sure no infection develops.

When to get help

Get help if the splinter is too deeply embedded into the skin to allow removal, or if the end of the splinter breaks off into the skin so you can't remove it. In the days following the removal of a splinter, look for signs of infection, such as reddening of the tissue, or a whitish-yellow area under the skin – which could indicate that pus is developing.

PREVENTION

 Use sandpaper to smooth rough edges of wooden furniture, fences, door-frames, etc.

 Keep children away from areas where metal or plastic cutting or shaving is taking place, or has already taken place.

 Check your home to see if there are any objects or furniture that might give your child a splinter.

Sprains – ligaments

See also Strains – pulled muscles.

A sprain is what happens when a ligament tears or gets over-stretched. A ligament is the fibrous tissue that holds the bones of a joint together. Gymnasts and dancers are very prone to this injury, and so are energetic and sporty children. The most usual place children get a sprain is in the ankle, as they make a sudden twist or slip sideways in their shoe. Sprains are caused by any type of pulling or wrenching movement, and are graded in terms of severity on a scale of 1 – 3, with 3 being the most serious.

Signs and symptoms

 mostly affects ankles, knees, wrists, shoulders, elbows

 pain and swelling in the affected area

 difficulty moving the area without increased pain

 tenderness when touched

 stiffness; cramps; bruising

 third-grade sprains – if the ligament has completely torn away from the bone, the joint can't hold the bones in place and the joint will be very wobbly

 if there is a tear, but the ligament is still attached, it is very painful but the joint is still stable

Method

After a sprain, the area should be rested. If the sprain is in the ankle or knee, raise your child's leg, as this will help reduce the flow of blood to the area and prevent further swelling. Apply an ice pack to the area or bathe with iced water – to help reduce the swelling. See 'Other care' below.

Cold compresses

Cold compresses will help to reduce the swelling.

Add the following essential oils to a bowl of water:

lavender – 3 drops
chamomile roman – 3 drops.

Put the compress in the water, squeeze it out, and apply to the area of the sprain.

Sprain (and strain) oil

For minor sprains, prepare the following mix:

1 dessertspoon vegetable oil
black pepper – 4 drops
ginger – 3 drops
helichrysum – 4 drops.

Smooth a small amount of the oil on to the affected area.

Over-8s sprain (and strain) oil

The following oil can be used on children over 8 years of age.

First, blend the following:

helichrysum – 20 drops
vegetable oil – 20 drops.

Use between 2 and 6 drops of this oil, depending on the size of the affected area. Put the oil directly on the sprain, three times a day – for two days only.

Essential oils that help

ginger
thyme linalol
lavender
chamomile roman
eucalyptus radiata
ormenis flower (chamomile maroc)
helichrysum
black pepper

Other care

Apply the physical and sports therapist's RICE rule – rest, ice, compression, elevation.

Rest   There should be no exercise until the area has healed.

 Ice   Crush ice in a plastic bag, wrap in a towel and apply to the area. Alternatively, freeze water in a polystyrene cup and, when it's frozen, cut the sides down slightly so there's a block you can apply directly on to the injured area. Apply the ice method for a few minutes, take the ice away for 5 minutes, then apply again.

 Compression   Wrap the area in an elastic bandage, making sure it supports the area, but is not so tight the area can't be moved, or the child's circulation is restricted. In the case of a shoulder, elbow or wrist, use a sling to restrict movement and to prevent further damage.

 Elevation   If the injury is in the ankle or knee, raise the injured area so it's higher than the heart.

When to get help

Get help if you suspect a fracture, if the bone looks out of shape or bent, or if the joint is wobbly. Also get help if your child is in a great deal of pain, even when the area is not being moved, or if after two days the area is more swollen, and painful to the touch.

PREVENTION

 Put your child in shoes that properly support the feet.

 If your child is sporty, ensure they wear trainers that are designed for the particular sport they do.

 Ensure that the sports equipment your child is using is of the correct size and weight for their body weight.

Strains – pulled muscles

See also Muscles – overexercised.

A strain refers to a tear or over-stretching of the muscular fibres or tendons. Strained muscles can occur anywhere in the body and are very painful. However, most strains are minor and will respond to home treatment and rest fairly quickly. The treatment for strains is similar, in some respects, to that for sprains – which is why in this section you will find similar information, and some references, to the *Sprains – pulled muscles* section.

Signs and symptoms

  pain and soreness in the muscle – hurts to move the area

  can affect anywhere – for example, stomach, limbs, neck

Method

Rest the strained area completely. If the strain is in the leg or arm, raise that limb to help reduce blood flow and reduce swelling in the area. Apply an ice pack to the area or bathe with iced water.

Cold compresses	Over-8s strain oil
Follow the instructions for the cold compress method in *Sprains – pulled muscles.*	Follow the instructions for the over-8s sprain (and strain) oil in *Sprains – pulled muscles.*

Strain oil 1

First, mix the following essential oils together:

ginger – 5 drops
black pepper – 2 drops
marjoram – 5 drops
ormenis flower (chamomile maroc) – 5 drops
helichrysum – 5 drops.

You now need to dilute a number of drops of this essential oil mix in 1 teaspoon vegetable oil. How many drops you need to use will depend on the age of your child – see page 27 for the 'general rule' guidelines.

When diluted, smooth the oil over the injured area. Then bandage the area, if the location of the strain makes that possible.

Strain oil 2

Follow the instructions for the sprain (and strain) oil in *Sprains – pulled muscles*.

Essential oils that help

ginger
thyme linalol
lavender
chamomile roman
eucalyptus radiata
ormenis flower (chamomile maroc)
helichrysum
black pepper

Other care

If the strain is in a muscle in an arm or leg, bandage the area to give support, making sure it's not too tight. Don't let your child exercise until the strained area has healed. Your child may benefit from the following natural remedies: Dr Bach's Rescue Remedy or Five Flower Essence Healing Herbs; homoeopathic arnica tablets; or Front Line Mother Essences.

When to get help

Get immediate medical help if your child experiences pain in an area of the body other than the area of the strain. Also, get help if your child is in severe pain that does not ease, or if swelling or inflammation develop. If, after 48 hours of resting, the strain does not appear to be improving, get medical advice.

PREVENTION

 As all dancers and athletes know, you should always stretch before exercising, and keep the muscles warm during and after exercise – tell your child this.

 Also tell your child not to try and push his or her body to achieve too much too soon – going at the right pace is important.

Stye

A stye is a bacterial infection that causes an inflamed, pus-filled sac on the edge of the upper or lower eyelid (often situated near the eyelashes). The stye can appear rather like a small boil, causing redness and swelling of the eyelid, which can make the eye seem almost closed. Styes can spread to other areas of the same eye, or from eye to eye, so hygiene is very important.

Signs and symptoms

 itchiness, soreness, redness and swelling of the eyelid

 becomes a lump under the skin, eventually turning into a pimple-type head of yellow pus

Method

Do not attempt to squeeze out the pus or remove it in any way – the body must be left to deal with the stye as best it can. Warm, wet compresses can give some relief, and help to soften the lump area, possibly bringing out the pus.

Essential oils that help

You cannot use any essential oils in the eye area. However, thoroughly sterilized essential oil hydrolats or 'waters' can be used in the compress or lid-bathing methods.

Hydrolat/'water' compress

First, turn to page 18 and read the section on hydrolats, so you are very clear about what these are. Boil the following together:

1 tablespoon lavender hydrolat
1 tablespoon chamomile hydrolat
2 tablespoons pure spring water
1 teaspoon witch hazel.

Allow to cool down.

When the mix is still slightly warm, put a small piece of muslin or similar light material in it. Squeeze out the excess liquid and lay the muslin over the closed eye.

Do this at least four times a day.

You can use the hyrolat/water mix above also to simply dab on the area of the stye – but only if you can avoid getting the mix into the eye itself. The child must be old enough to understand that they must keep the eye tightly shut. Don't use cotton wool to dab the area, because little bits may get into the eye and irritate it even further.

Filter method of compress

First, turn to page 18 and read the section on hydrolats and 'waters', so you are very clear about what these are.

1 tablespoon rose water
1 tablespoon chamomile hydrolat/'water' chamomile roman – 1 drop
2 tablespoons pure spring water
1 teaspoon witch hazel.

Heat the above ingredients, then pour through an unbleached paper coffee-filter.

Do not forget the paper-filter part of these instructions.

When cooled, use in the compress method – dipping muslin in the liquid mix, squeezing it out well and applying over the stye area. The eye must be tightly closed, so this can only be used with children who can be trusted to do that.

You can also use the mix above to dab on the area of the stye – but only if you can avoid getting it into the eye itself. Don't use cotton wool.

Cheek oil

This oil is for putting on the cheekbone. Do not put it anywhere around the eye at all. Apply very little – just dab. Wipe off any excess with a tissue straight away.

Mix together:

$1/2$ teaspoon vegetable oil
lavender – 5 drops.

Apply only a tiny amount with a fingertip along the cheekbone.

Other care

The stye will disappear without any help, around five days after the pus has gone. Unfortunately, new ones often appear, close to the original site. Some children are very prone to styes, and good nutrition is important for them.

When to get help

Get medical advice if the redness and swelling carry on for a long time, if the stye seems to be getting worse or doesn't seem to be disappearing, if there are a cluster of styes, or if the stye is still there after one month.

Sunburn

See also Heat exhaustion; Heatstroke.

Sunburn is caused by too much exposure to the ultraviolet rays of the sun, in combination with not wearing enough protection. Sunburn can be very uncomfortable and is serious in the case of babies and infants, whose skin is thinner than an older child's or adult's. Repeated sunburn in young children can lead to more serious problems in later life.

Signs and symptoms

 redness or pinkness of the skin

 skin feels sore when touched

 sometimes with swelling and blistering

 sunburn can take 24 hours after exposure to reach its worst

fever is sometimes present

 the dead, dried skin can start to peel away after about three days

Method

The worst thing you can do is to try and peel away the skin if it starts to peel. Let it come off in its own time, no matter how unsightly it is. Cool baths help a lot, especially immediately after exposure to the sun. On areas that aren't submerged in baths – the face and neck – use cold compresses.

Baths

Run a cool bath, and add neat lavender essential oil according to the age of the child:
5 years – 3 drops
6 years – 4 drops
7 years – 5 drops
8 years – 6 drops.

The older your child is, add 1 extra drop per year – to a maximum of 12 drops.

If any lavender gets into the eyes, it will sting, so make sure your child is aware they should not splash about. If your child is young, stay with them to make sure they don't splash.

Compresses

To 30 ml (1 ounce) water, add 5 drops lavender essential oil. Swish the water around. Soak the compress material in this, then squeeze it out.

If you place the compress over the face, make sure your child keeps their eyes closed. The eyelids often get sunburned. For this, you could soak cotton-wool balls in the compress water, making sure you really squeeze them out well, and place over the eye, like eyepads. Stay with your child to make sure that they do not open their eyes.

Repeat the compress or cotton-wool ball methods as often as you can.

Hydrolat compress

If you have lavender or chamomile hydrolats (or 'waters'), use them in the compress method. Soak the compress material in the hydrolat – either lavender or chamomile, or a combination of both. Squeeze out, and place gently over the burned areas of skin.

Prepare a lot of compresses and keep them in the refrigerator. Use them throughout the day, until the child's skin has cooled down.

This method is particularly helpful in cases of sunburn on the face or eyelids – but make sure the child's eyes are closed.

Aloe vera

The aloe vera plant is used all over the world to soothe the skin after too much exposure to the sun. The plant grows easily and doesn't take much looking after, and you can cut a leaf any time to extract the gooey healing juice inside the thick, hard leaves.

Mix together:

1 teaspoon aloe vera
lavender – 5 drops.

Smear the mixture over sunburned skin.

Calamine lotion

Calamine lotion is readily available, and essential oil can be added to it. Mix together:

250 ml (8 ounces) calamine lotion
chamomile german – 10 drops
lavender – 30 drops.

Shake the bottle well, and apply to affected areas.

Essential oils that help

lavender
chamomile german
eucalyptus radiata

Other care

See 'Prevention' below.

When to get help

Get medical help if the skin is very sore, or if it's blistering. Also get medical help if your child has a headache or other pain, a temperature, dry mouth, or if they are shivering.

PREVENTION

It's important to use common sense when going out in the sun with children.

 Don't take young children and infants in the sun without high-factor sunscreen, sunhats and other protective clothing, and a sunshade.

 Sunscreen should not be used on babies less than six months old, so make sure your baby is kept out of the sunlight and wears appropriate protective clothing.

 Put sunscreen on all children in any strong sunlight. Keep all children out of strong sun between 11 a.m. and 2 p.m.

 Take adequate clothing when going in the sun, including a hat, and T-shirt to wear at the beach or swimming pool.

 Make sure your child drinks often if they are in the sun.

After being in the sun, even if there is no redness on the skin, put a cooling lotion, gel or plain water on your child's body, in order to cool it down.

 Teach your child the rules about going in the sun, no matter what colour skin your child has – Caucasian, Asian, Afro-American or mixed race. All skins can burn.

'Swimmer's ear' (external otitis)

'Swimmer's ear' (or external otitis) is an inflammation in the visible part of the ear canal, caused by a bacterial or fungal infection, which is caught while swimming. It's less common in swimming pools that use chlorine and other chemical products in the water. But it's common in lakes, especially during the summer, and can also be found in the ocean. External otitis can also be caught through poor hygiene – if a child touches bacteria with his or her hands and inserts fingers or other objects into the ears. Once a child has the infection, further outbreaks seem to be more likely.

Signs and symptoms

 redness in ear; itching; pain

 fluid coming out of the ear

Method

Ear ointment

Mix the following together thoroughly:

15 ml ($^1/_2$ ounce) vegetable-based (Vaseline-type) ointment
chamomile german – 10 drops
thyme linalol – 4 drops
palmarosa – 4 drops.

Apply a small amount to the outer ear canal.

To make an earplug, put a little ointment on a large piece of cotton wool (much larger than the ear-hole). Tuck it in the ear, and leave there for at least an hour.

A tiny amount of the anti-bacterial mix (page 49) can be smeared around the ear to help stem the infection.

Essential oils that help

thyme linalol
chamomile german
palmarosa

When to get help

Get medical help if there is pain or discharge from the ear, if the ear seems swollen, or if your child scratches his or her ears a lot.

PREVENTION

 Don't swim in lake water if it looks murky, when the weather is very hot and humid, or if you've heard that other people have caught infections or rashes from that lake.

Before your child goes swimming, gently wipe a tiny amount of olive oil or vegetable-based (Vaseline-type) ointment around the outer part of the ear and ear canal.

 Have your child wear earplugs, or pull a swimming hat down over the ears.

 Dry the ears thoroughly after each swim (wherever that happens to be) and, if there are showers, use them.

Swollen lymph glands/nodes

See also Mononucleosis; Sore throat.

When a gland in the neck or groin swells, it means that it's fighting an infection and really doing its job. The first sign of infection is often when the lymph nodes swell up; other symptoms then follow. The lymph nodes act as a filter system, preventing bacteria, viruses and other micro-organisms from entering the bloodstream. Sometimes the lymph nodes themselves become infected, preceding an infection.

Signs and symptoms

 glands in the neck or groin area swell, and feel very sore and painful when touched

 glands in neck: throat seems red and swollen

Method

Lymph gland oil

A swollen lymph node can be large and hard, or small and pea-like. Certain essential oils applied to this area will have a good chance of dealing with the infection, such as thyme linalol and tea tree.

For children 6 and over, apply 1 drop neat essential oil (either of the above) directly on the swollen lymph node – in the neck or in the groin area (being careful to avoid the genitals). If two glands are swollen, put 1 drop on each.

Do this twice a day, for no longer than three days.

For children 5 years and under, dilute the drop of essential oil with 1 drop vegetable oil, then apply as above.

Compresses

Use the compress method in the usual way, using lukewarm water and the following essential oils:

thyme linalol – 6 drops
tea tree – 5 drops.

Soak in the water, squeeze out well and apply over the swollen area.

Essential oils that help

Different essential oils help, depending on the particular infection. Without knowing which particular bacteria or organism has infected your child, advice cannot be given. However, in the following list the stronger anti-bacterials come first.

thyme linalol
tea tree
manuka
lavender
chamomile german
chamomile roman

Other care

The plant echinacea is very useful at fighting infection, and comes in different preparations (always follow the directions on the packet). Drops are far easier to take than the tablet form, especially for children, and are more easily absorbed. Increase your child's intake of vitamin C.

When to get help

Get help if there is a temperature or fever, sore throat, stiff neck, or rash. Get emergency medical help if there is a swelling in one of the glands in the body (with no pain) that doesn't go away after two weeks, and there's weight loss, night sweats, tiredness, bruising or a small, reddish-purple rash. This group of symptoms could indicate lymphoma.

Tattooing

Human beings have been tattooing themselves since earliest historic times – despite the fact that it's sometimes difficult to understand why they should want to do it. Today, tattoos are a major fashion statement, with girls as well as boys, pre-teens as well as teenagers and young adults. Basically, tattooing is the insertion of permanent colour under the surface of the skin with the use of needles. Problems with infection do occasionally occur when the job is done professionally, but trouble can really start when juveniles decide that it's something they can do to each other.

Tattooing is not without its risks. Unsterilized equipment may transmit not only viral, bacterial and fungal infection, but tetanus, hepatitis and HIV. Problems can also arise if there is an allergic reaction to the chemicals in the dye or ink used.

Few parents are pleased when their child comes home with a tattoo, but, rather than getting highly emotional over it, take precautionary measures to ensure your child's safety. It's important to find out under what circumstances the tattooing was done – ask whether the needles were sterilized, and how it was done. If you feel there may be a major risk, consult your doctor. In other cases, apply the measures below.

If infection has already occurred, you must visit your doctor because of the risks involved. In adulthood, dermabrasion and laser treatment can be used to remove tattoos, but they usually leave some degree of scarring.

Method

To help prevent infection

First, wash the area with a strong disinfectant solution. Then, mix together:

thyme linalol – 20 drops
lavender – 20 drops
tea tree – 20 drops.

From this blend of neat essential oils, apply 1 drop over each square inch of the affected area, to a maximum of 5 drops. Leave to dry.

Repeat as often as possible over the coming week.

Essential oils that help

These oils help infection on tattooed areas:

thyme linalol
manuka
lavender
niaouli
tea tree
elemi
chamomile german

Parent's tip

If your child has been pressurized at school into having a tattoo and doesn't really want it, try wiping the area with neat lemon, orange or grapefruit essential oil. These oils can cause skin irritation. Also, they are photosensitive and the skin shouldn't be exposed to sunlight while the oils are on it. But, if used directly after home tattooing, these citrus oils often help to fade the markings (if not available, try lemon juice).

Teething

Babies usually start teething from the age of 6 months; by the time they're 2 years of age, twenty 'milk' teeth will have emerged from the gums. Some teeth will have difficulty coming through, and will cause soreness and pain. To find out if your child is teething, look to see if there are inflamed areas on the gum and, with a very clean finger, feel around the gums for hard bumps. If you find either of these things, the likelihood is that baby is teething.

271

Signs and symptoms

 dribbling; rashes around the mouth

 biting on anything; baby trying to put fist in the mouth

 possible fever or runny stools

 difficulty sleeping; crying; irritability

Method

Above all, at this time, babies need reassuring with cuddles and comfort. Adopt the classic pose of a parent with a teething child – walking up and down, patting his or her back, saying 'There, there'.

Cool compress

Apply a cool compress over the jaw area, made using

lavender hydrolat/'water'
chamomile hydrolat/'water'.

(See page 18 for how hydrolats or essential oil 'waters' are made.)

Dip a folded piece of muslin into the hydrolat or 'water', squeeze it out well, and place it along baby's jawline.

Oil to help sleep

First, mix the following together:

I dessertspoon vegetable oil
petitgrain – I drop
lavender – I drop.

Rub a small amount of the diluted oil over the back, the back of the neck and the soles of the feet.

Essential oils that help

chamomile german
chamomile roman
cardamom
eucalyptus radiata

Essential oils that help for calming and sleep

lavender
petitgrain

Other care

Homeopathic 'chamomile teething' granules may help. Give your child soothing, soft, cool, foods such as yoghurt, ice cream and jelly. Teething rings help the soreness – but keep them in the refrigerator, not the freezer. If you give your baby peeled apple or carrot to gnaw on, make sure you stay in the same room.

When to get help

Get help if your baby has any symptoms that concern you.

Threadworms (Enterobius vermicularis)

This is a very common parasitic infection, usually found in children between the ages of 5 and 9. The worms are about 1 cm (^{1}/2 inch) long and thin, and resemble pieces of white cotton. They live in the child's intestines and usually come out at night, often causing the child to wake up and complain of itching around the anal or vulval area.

The eggs can easily be passed from person to person. Although the eggs can be breathed in through the air, the most usual way for a child to become infected is by handling toilet seats, toys and other contaminated objects, and then putting their fingers in their mouths.

Essential oils can be used as a complementary treatment to the medication available through your doctor or chemist. Baths are often recommended as a way of helping to soothe the anal area.

Signs and symptoms

 itching around the buttocks or anus, and sometimes the vagina – especially shortly after going to bed; disturbed sleep

 red, irritated skin around the anus

 white, threadlike worms in the stools

 irritability; child seems generally unwell

 threadworms and other parasites may be responsible for weight loss; swollen abdomen; inability to concentrate; lethargy; headaches; and teeth-grinding

Essential oils that help

niaouli
fennel
lavender
cardamom
chamomile roman
clove
bay

Method

Tummy massage

Use for no longer than one week.

Into 30 ml (1 ounce) sesame seed oil, mix the following:

clove – 3 drops   niaouli – 6 drops
cardamom – 10 drops   bay – 8 drops.

Rub a small amount of the mix over the child's back and stomach area. Cover with a warm, dry compress until cool. Then massage a small amount of plain sesame oil over the stomach only.

Soothing lotion

To help soothe the area, bathe the anus with a small amount of the following lotion. First, mix together:

15 ml ($^{1}/_{2}$ ounce) aloe vera gel
15 ml ($^{1}/_{2}$ ounce) chamomile water
15 ml ($^{1}/_{2}$ ounce) lavender water.

Then add:
lavender – 2 drops
cardamom – 1 drop.

Mix well, and soothe a small amount around the anus after being to the toilet.

Baths

In 1 teaspoon vegetable oil, mix the following:

cardamom – 4 drops
chamomile roman – 3 drops.

Use $^{1}/_{4}$ teaspoon in a bath for children between 5 and 7 years, and $^{1}/_{2}$ teaspoon for older children.

Other care

Use medication available from your doctor or chemist.

Give the child plenty of cabbage, onions and garlic, and get him or her to drink pomegranate juice frequently.

Herbal tinctures such as black walnut are available in health food shops.

The worms come out of the body to lay their eggs, so, to encourage the worms to come out of the body, get your child to sit in a bowl of warm milk (which will attract the worms). If your child can be made to pass faeces at this time, all the better; do this after medication has been taken. Read to your child to distract attention from what is happening. Afterwards, wash the child's bottom in soap and warm water.

PREVENTION

 Teach children to wash their hands thoroughly with soap after going to the bathroom, and before snacks and mealtimes.

 Put a couple of drops of essential oil on tissues and wipe over toilet seats.

 When using public toilets, teach girls to pass urine while slightly standing so they don't actually touch the toilet seat.

 To discourage airborne eggs, use the spray method (which puts a fine mist of essential oils in the air).

Thrush (Candida albicans – 'yeast infection')

See also Nappy rash.

Yeasts are a type of fungus. *Candida albicans* (a yeast/fungal infection) can flourish almost anywhere within the gastrointestinal tract of babies, children and adults, and can infect the mouth, throat, stomach, intestines, anus, and (in girls) the vaginal and vulval area. Sometimes this yeast/fungal infection is called 'thrush' or 'candidiasis'.

Babies can catch thrush during labour from their mother's birth canal, or it can be caught anytime afterwards from infected nipples or feeding bottles. Children who have general low resistance are at risk, as are those who have been on long courses of antibiotics – which not only kill off targeted unfriendly bacteria, but also the normal 'friendly' bacteria that live in a healthy intestinal tract. When there are no longer enough 'friendly' bacteria to fight off the yeast infection, the infection is left free to become rampant.

Signs and symptoms

 whitish, cream-coloured frothy creamy patches on the roof of the mouth, gums, inner cheeks, tongue, and sometimes the lips

 child may refuse to eat

 creamy patches around the anus and (in girls) possibly around the vaginal and vulval area

 rash similar to nappy rash; pimple-filled red patch

 rash spots can cause sores if the outer, white coating is rubbed off

Baths

If the genital area has become infected, use the other methods (above) and, when your child has a bath, add 1 teaspoon of bicarbonate of soda to the water.

Essential oils that help

tea tree
manuka
chamomile german
palmarosa
thyme linalol
geranium
patchouli

Method

Anal washing

Use either of the methods below, to help keep infection and irritation in the area under control.

Yoghurt method
Stir together well:

**30 ml (1 ounce) carton of plain, unflavoured, bioactive yoghurt
tea tree – 5 drops
chamomile german – 3 drops
palmarosa – 5 drops.**

Use a tiny amount to spread around the anal area – after each nappy change, or after using the toilet.

'Tea' wash method
See page 54 for instructions on how to make an essential oil 'tea'.

Prepare a 'tea', using:

**$^1/_2$ pint water
tea tree – 5 drops
palmarosa – 5 drops**

chamomile german – 5 drops.

Use the 'tea' to wash or wipe the anal area – after each nappy change, or after using the toilet. Bioactive natural yoghurt can also be added to this tea.

Body oil

The following mix can be diluted in vegetable oil to make a body oil. Use it over the whole body, avoiding the face and genital area.

See page 9 for instructions on how many drops of the mix to use, depending on the age of your child.

First, mix together:

tea tree – 10 drops
chamomile german – 6 drops
palmarosa – 6 drops.

Mouthwash

Only use this method if your child's mouth is affected, and with children who are old enough to use a mouthwash and spit it out afterwards.

See page 54 for instructions on how to make an essential oil 'tea'.

Prepare a 'tea', using:

$^1/_2$ pint water
tea tree – I drop
palmarosa – I drop
chamomile german – I drop.

Now pour the 'tea' through an unbleached paper coffee-filter and bottle.

To prepare the mouthwash, mix together:

I dessertspoon filtered 'tea'
$^1/_4$ pint water
I dessertspoon unflavoured bioactive yoghurt.

Have your child use this as a mouthwash, making sure he or she spits it out afterwards.

Other care

To stop the infection spreading from the mouth to the genital area, and vice versa, make sure your child washes hands before and after going to the toilet. If your child is a baby, leave his or her nappy off as much as possible.

Give your infant cool foods to help soothe the mouth. The best choice would be unflavoured, unsweetened, bioactive yoghurt – the type that has active 'friendly' bacteria in it. Avoid all products that contain sugar, as the fungus thrives on a diet of sugar. Get older children to avoid eating dairy produce, wheat products, and foods containing yeast. Consider giving your child acidophilus supplements. See also 'Prevention' below.

When to get help

Get help as soon as you suspect your child has thrush.

PREVENTION

See 'Other care' above.

Good hygiene is essential in order to help prevent your baby being infected with thrush.

 Before feeding your baby from the breast, wash the nipple area. If going out and about, take an antispetic wipe with you, and use it to clean the nipple before placing it in baby's mouth.

 If you bottle-feed your baby, wash your hands before preparing feeds. Make sure you first boil, then sterilize, all bottle teats.

 Public bathrooms sometimes provide nappy-changing facilities. However, this is not the ideal place to feed your baby, as bacteria from faecal matter can be airborne.

Tonsillitis

See also Sore throat.

Tonsillitis is an inflammation of the tonsils – two patches on either side of the throat, right at the back, which can be seen when the child opens his or her mouth very wide. As part of the lymphatic system, the job of the tonsils is to help fight infection by trapping germs and preventing them from entering the respiratory system and other parts of the body. The tonsils often become enlarged when a child is fighting an infection.

Tonsillitis is usually caused by the bacteria streptococcus but sometimes by a virus, and the adenoids may also become infected. It is more common in children of school age.

Signs and symptoms

 sore throat; difficulty in swallowing

 tonsils seem red – inflammation; may have white spots of pus on them

 temperature may go over 37.7° C (100° F)

 possible bad breath; snoring during sleep

 possible headache; earache; neckache; tummy ache

 possible chills; cough

Method

To see if your child's tonsils are infected, open his or her mouth wide and hold the tongue down with a tongue depressor or the back of a spoon handle. Tell your child to say 'Aaah' – this way you'll be able to see more of the throat. Check your child's temperature, and feel either side of the neck to see if the glands are swollen.

Gargle

This method can only be used by children who are old enough to gargle and spit out afterwards. Use only 1 teaspoon in a glass of warm water for a gargle.

First, mix together:

30 ml (1 ounce) pure spring water
3 tablespoons cider vinegar
ginger – 3 drops
lemon – 5 drops.

Stir everything together, then pour through an unbleached paper coffee-filter. Then mix in:

1 tablespoon honey.

Stir the honey in well, until the liquid is all one consistency, then bottle.

Put 1 teaspoon of the final mix in a small glass of warm water, and use as a gargle. Do this twice a day.

Glands oil

Put a couple of drops of pure thyme linalol essential oil on your fingertips and apply over the glands on either side of the neck. Then gently wipe a little vegetable oil over the top. Repeat before sleep every night.

Tonsillitis compress and oil mix

This mix was published in one of my earlier books (*The Fragrant Pharmacy*) and I know from the many letters I've received that it's been very effective. This is a two-part method.

First, mix the essential oils together:

lavender – 10 drops
tea tree – 15 drops
ginger – 5 drops
lemon – 2 drops.

Warm compress
Use 4 drops of the tonsillitis mix above in the compress method. Put warm water in a bowl, add the essential oils, put a cloth in the water, squeeze it out, and place it over the throat area.

Do this twice a day.

Abdomen and back oil
Mix together:

1 dessertspoon vegetable oil
tonsillitis mix - 5 drops.

Using a small amount each time, apply over the upper abdomen and upper back.

Rose syrup

This syrup goes down a treat when the tonsils are sore. This is what you will need:

enough fragrant, organically grown rose petals to fill a pint jar
1lb organic brown granulated sugar
1 pint spring water
juice of 1 lemon
rose otto – 3 drops.

First, wash the rose petals thoroughly in water.

Put the spring water, with the rose petals, into a small cooking pot. Cover the pot with a lid and bring to the boil. Turn the heat down, so the pot can simmer very gently for 10 minutes. Then turn the heat off completely, but leave the pot right where it is, for another two hours.

Strain the mixture, then top up the water level until it's back to 1 pint again. Then add the lemon juice, the essential oil drops and the sugar. Stir slowly until it thickens, then pour into jars.

Honey is very soothing for all types of sore throat. The above method can be used, substituting 1lb honey for the 1lb sugar. Use very thick-set honey.

Essential oils that help

lavender
tea tree
thyme linalol
lemon
ginger
chamomile roman
chamomile german

Other care

Give your child soothing drinks. Use warm compresses over the throat area. Keep the air circulating in your child's room.

When to get help

If your child is a small baby, contact your doctor as soon as you suspect tonsillitis. With all other children, get medical help if your child can't swallow properly, if they have a high fever, complain of earache, or if the condition generally seems to be getting worse.

Toothache

Pain in the teeth area can be caused by tooth decay, gum infection, biting on a hard object, or an injury to a tooth.

Signs and symptoms

 pain in the tooth or gum

 earache

 a tooth problem can be felt as face-ache; the face may become swollen (often a sign of an abscess)

 drinking or eating something cold, hot or sweet causes pain (a sign of tooth decay)

 red and swollen gums (a sign of an abscess or gumboil)

Jaw oil

Mix together the following:

1 teaspoon vegetable oil
clove – 1 drop
helichrysum – 1 drop
chamomile german – 3 drops.

Rub a little of the diluted oil along the external jawline.

Compresses

Use warm water or, if the child prefers it, ice-cold water.

Put 30 ml (1 ounce) water in a small bowl, and add:

chamomile roman – 2 drops.

Soak the compress material in the water, squeeze out, and apply to the painful side of the jaw.

Mouth rinses and rubs

Only use this method with children over 5 years of age. The child must be able to rinse the mouth then spit the liquid out. Use tincture of myrrh (available from chemists) and follow directions on the packaging.

For infected gums, make your own myrrh tincture by adding 2 drops of myrrh essential oil to 1 teaspoon consumable alcohol, such as brandy or vodka, and 1 dessertspoon water. Put it all into a dropper bottle. When ready for use, put just one drop of the mix into 1 teaspoon warm water. Dip a cotton-wool bud into this, and use it to rub gently around the gum. Use a clean bud each time.

If gumboils are present, add 1 drop of thyme linalol to the above mix.

Essential oils that help

chamomile roman
chamomile german
clove
helichrysum
lemon
myrrh

Other care

Ice packs or cold compresses may help reduce the swelling. Pain can sometimes be relieved by warmth applied to the area – such as in warm compresses, or by a warm towel or hot-water bottle being held against the affected side of the face. Check the lymph glands to see if they are swollen (see *Swollen lymph glands/nodes*, page 267).

When to get help

Consult your dentist to prevent tooth decay and other problems. See your doctor if there has been any facial injury.

PREVENTION

　Regular visits to the dentist will help identify any potential problems.

　Teach your child to brush his or her teeth correctly, and to floss after eating and before bedtime. Visit a dental hygienist, who can teach your child proper tooth-care habits.

　Cut down on intake of sweets, sweet foods and drinks.

　Give your child water to drink after eating sweets, to flush through the sugar.

Do not give young children bottles of juice at bedtime – even pure fruit juice. After the child's teeth have been brushed, only give water.

 Give drinks to small children in a plastic beaker-type cup with a lid, and a mouthpiece that is long enough to bypass the teeth area.

Tuberculosis (TB)

Although rare, TB is on the increase. It's caused by the Mycobacterium tuberculosis bacterium, and used to be spread through the milk of infected cows, but these days it's usually caught by breathing in the droplets put into the atmosphere by infected people coughing or sneezing. TB mostly affects the lungs, but can involve all the organs of the body when spread through the bloodstream. There are various forms of TB, which can be identified by a simple skin test.

Signs and symptoms

 there may be no symptoms except flu-like symptoms (which are often mistaken for flu); children with recurrent bouts of flu should be checked for TB

 persistent dry cough

 nighttime sweating

 possible blood in the sputum

 chest pain

 headache; lack of appetite; lack of energy; weight loss; fever

Method

Tuberculosis (TB) mix

This mix can be used in the two methods below. Follow the instructions in each box. First, mix the following essential oils together:

thyme linalol – 10 drops
ravensara – 10 drops
niaouli – 10 drops.

Body oil
From the TB mix above, take double the number of drops recommended for your child's age on page 27, and add to 30 ml (1 ounce) vegetable oil.

Use the oil to rub over the whole of your child's body, twice a day. This amount will be enough for several applications, depending on the size of your child.

Warm baths
From the TB mix above, take the number of drops recommended for your child's age on page 27, and add to 1 teaspoon vegetable oil.

Put in the bath water, and swish around well before your child gets in.

Essential oils that help

ravensara
niaouli
thyme linalol
eucalyptus radiata

In diffuser or other room methods only
oregano
cinnamon
clove

Other care

Your child will need plenty of rest, and a good diet of home cooking, with a multivitamin supplement. Your child may have to be absent from school for several months, so keep him or her occupied with home-study activities by liaising with his or her teacher. Your child will not be infectious once drug treatment from your doctor has been started; then they can play with other children.

When to get help

Inform your doctor as soon as possible if any of the above symptoms occur. Get medical advice if your child has been in the company of anyone with TB.

PREVENTION

   Inoculations are available.

   A skin test can determine whether your child has TB.

Umbilical cord infection

At birth, the umbilical cord is clamped and cut, and over the next seven to ten days the remaining stump shrivels up, then falls off. It can become infected if cleaning is not carried out correctly, or if urine or faecal matter have seeped into the area.

Signs and symptoms

   redness and swelling together

   fluid weeping from the stump

crusting over; pus

 after the cord drops off, discharge from the area (a sign of infection)

Method

Cleaning methods

Newborn babies have very thin skin, as it has yet to mature. Only use very small amounts of anything on newborn skin.

Cleansing wash
First, put 1 drop of lavender oil into 1 teaspoon salt, and add to the water you are going to use for washing. Then, pour through an unbleached paper coffee-filter. Now use to bathe the area gently.

Cotton-wool bud method
First wash your hands. Put 1 drop of lavender oil on to a cotton-wool bud. Dip the bud in a cup of water, squeeze the excess water out between your fingertips. Use the bud to clean carefully around the area. Do this twice a day.

Neat oil

Use this method if your baby's umbilical cord clearly has signs of infection. First wash your hands. Smear a tiny amount of neat lavender oil (less than 1 drop) on one of your fingertips, and wipe that fingertip in a circle around the base of the stump, taking care not to touch any infected or cut area.

Essential oils that help

tea tree
lavender
chamomile german

Other care

Wipe the cord after each nappy change. Some people recommend using surgical spirit. Use a little salt water in baby's bath, and also bathe the affected area with salt water. Always let the stump fall off naturally, so a nice belly button is formed.

When to get help

Get help if the stump seems red or swollen, or if there is a discharge.

PREVENTION

 Always check the cord stump at each nappy change.

 As often as possible, leave the umbilical area exposed to the air. This helps it dry up.

Urinary tract infection

Urinary tract infection is usually caused by bacteria in the urinary system, but can also be caused by viral or fungal infection. It can affect the kidneys, ureter, bladder and urethra. Cystitis is the most common type of urinary tract infection, but there are others, such as urethritis and pyelonephritis.

Signs and symptoms

 can occur in girls and boys; often occurs in uncircumcised male children

 burning sensation when passing urine

 strongly coloured urine; strong-smelling urine

 feeling the frequent need of urination, often with just a dribble

 back pain may be located just above the waistline

 possible tummy pain; nauseous feeling; vomiting

 in children who were previously dry at night – bed-wetting (as the body tries to rid itself of the infection)

Method

Warm baths

Dilute 3 drops of tea tree oil in 1 teaspoon vegetable oil, and add to the warm bath water. Also add 1 teaspoon salt to the water. Swish around well before the child gets in.

Urinary tract mix

The following mix can be used in the three methods below. Follow the directions in each box. First mix the following together:

niaouli – 5 drops
tea tree – 5 drops
bergamot – 5 drops
mandarin – 5 drops
chamomile german – 6 drops.

Warm compresses
Apply warm compresses over your child's back, just above the waistline.

Put ¹/₂ pint warm water in a bowl and add:

5 drops of the 'Urinary tract mix' (above).

Soak the compress material in the water, squeeze out, and apply.

Body oil for the back
See page 9 for the number of drops of essential oil to use for your child's age, in the 'body rub' method.

Use the appropriate number of drops of the 'Urinary tract mix' (above), diluted in the appropriate amount of vegetable oil.

Gently rub over the lower back.

Boys' wash
Put the following in a clean bowl:

¹/₂ pint lukewarm water
1 teaspoon salt
'Urinary tract mix' (above) - 5 drops.

Swish the water around well, and use to bathe the penis. Gently pull back the foreskin and wash the area underneath.

Essential oils that help

tea tree
bergamot
niaouli
lavender
chamomile german

Other care

Give your child plenty of pure, unadulterated cranberry juice, as this helps to clear up urinary infection. Freeze-dried powdered cranberry can be used by older children. If no cranberry juice is available, buy frozen cranberries and cook them in water. Then put the fruit and cooking water into a liquidizer, adding enough additional water to make a juice. Sieve the juice before giving it to your child. Do not add sugar at any point in the process.

Increase your child's water intake: he or she must not be given any fizzy or sugar-laden drinks. Don't let the child use bubble bath or other bath preparations – only use diluted essential oils. Put your child in pure cotton underwear. Warm compresses, hot-water bottles or warm towels placed over the kidney area often helps – apply on the back, just above the waist.

When to get help

Get medical help if your child complains of pain when passing urine, if the urine smells unusually unpleasant, is cloudy or very strongly coloured. Also get help if your child is itchy in the area, or feels the need to pass urine frequently, but cannot do so.

PREVENTION

 Teach girls that, after urinating, they should wipe from the front of the genital area towards the back.

Vomiting

See also Dehydration.

When food or fluid is regurgitated from the stomach, it's called vomiting. Vomiting is one of the ways the body rids itself of infection or toxins that have entered the body, usually in the form of a bacteria or other micro-organisms. If the vomiting is serious, it can lead to dehydration.

Babies and infants often regurgitate their food, and this is nothing to worry about. But when a child of any age has what's known as projectile vomiting, there is something to worry about. This is when food or liquid is thrown up with such force that it lands several feet away. Projectile vomiting is caused by a muscular abnormality, and must be seen by a doctor as soon as possible. Insist that your child is given a thorough examination.

Sign and symptom

 uncontrollable regurgitation of food or liquid through the mouth

Method

Vomiting mix

Use the following essential oils in equal amounts in the two methods below:

lavender
cardamom.

Compresses
Use only on children over 2.

Put I pint of cool or lukewarm water in a bowl, and add 2 drops each of lavender and cardamom essential oil. Swish around well. Put a cloth in the water and squeeze it out well. Ask your child to close his or her eyes, then place the compress over the forehead.

Tissue or pillow
Mix together a couple of drops of lavender and cardamom essential oil, using equal amounts. Use one of these methods:

Put I drop of the mix on a tissue and give it to your child to sniff.

Put I drop on your child's pillow – on the underside, away from the eyes. Lay your child down to rest. The essential oils will calm your child if he or she is fretful, and help the child to fall asleep.

Essential oils that help

cardamom
ginger
peppermint
spearmint
lavender

Other care

Do not attempt to stop the vomiting. When your child is vomiting, hold the forehead steady, and pull hair out of the way. After each bout of vomiting, wash your child's face gently with cool or lukewarm water. You could also place a cool wet flannel or a compress over your child's forehead or on the back of the neck – this cools the child down and generally makes him or her feel better.

Give your child nothing to eat or drink until at least one hour after the vomiting has stopped. Then give a small glass of cooled-down boiled water, and ask your child to take small sips continuously.

When to get help

Get help immediately if there are stomach cramps, fever, headache, coughing, or if the vomiting continues for longer than five hours.

PREVENTION

 Don't try to prevent vomiting. It's best to let the body rid itself of whatever it needs to.

Warts

Warts are caused by the human papillomavirus, and are benign skin growths. They have to be transmitted by direct contact, and can be contracted in public places if someone touches a surface after an infected person has touched it. There are several types, including: hand warts, the so-called 'plantar' warts (which attach themselves to feet), and 'flat' warts that grow on the face.

Sexually active teenagers are at risk of genital warts, which can appear on the penis or vulval area. Girls with genital warts are at risk of cervical cancer, and genital warts (in boys as well as in girls) must be treated immediately by a doctor.

Signs and symptoms

 Hand warts   These grow on the child's hand or fingers – usually on the back of the hand, the fingers, and around the fingernail. They start out as small bumps, often pinkish in colour. They're elevated above the surface of the flesh, and have a scaly surface. Sometimes there's a horn-type of protrusion. These often disappear all by themselves in time.

 Plantar warts   Plantar warts grow on the feet, and the infection is often picked up walking around swimming pools, gyms and showers. The wart has a central core, which starts out soft but gradually grows into a hard, horny surface area, level with the flesh. They have a distinct core, which is often marked by a black spot. This spot is made up of blood vessels.

 Flat warts   Flat warts can grow on a child's face, and are 'flat' because they are much smoother than other types of wart and are close to the surface of the skin. Although generally smaller than other types of wart, they can grow in groups of as many as 20. Facial warts should only be treated by a doctor.

Method

The following recommendations are only for warts on the hand and fingers, or plantar warts on the feet or toes.

Hand, finger, foot and toe wart mix

Use this mix in either of the two methods below.

First, mix the following essential oils together:

lemon – 10 drops
bergamot – 5 drops
cypress – 2 drops
manuka – 5 drops
thyme red – 4 drops
clove – 1 drop.

Hand and finger warts
This method can only be used if your child can be guaranteed not to put his or her hand anywhere near their mouth or face.

Dip a clean cotton-wool bud into the wart mix, and dab a small amount of the mix directly on the wart. Use only once a day, for no more than 10 days.

Plantar warts – feet and toes
Dip a clean cotton-wool bud into the wart mix, and dab a small amount of the mix directly on the wart. Do this twice a day, for no more than 10 days.

Essential oils that help

lemon
bergamot
cypress
manuka
thyme linalol
Dermatect (see 'Suppliers')

When to get help

Get help if the wart is bleeding, or if your child is scratching the wart and there's a risk of infection. Take advice if the wart doesn't disappear after eight weeks. Also, get help if the wart is swollen or becomes red or if for any reason either you or the child are worried. A doctor can freeze the warts.

Whooping cough

Whooping cough is a highly contagious disease caused by the *Bordetella pertussis* bacterium. It affects the respiratory system, with the airways becoming blocked with mucus. The most characteristic symptom is a high-pitched 'whoop' sound made as the air tries to pass through a swollen larynx during a coughing bout. Whooping cough can last up to eight weeks, during which time the child is especially vulnerable to bronchitis or pneumonia (see pages 90 and 222), as well as other serious conditions.

Signs and symptoms

   starts with cold-like symptoms that last 10–14 days, then the cough starts

   cough – with or without the 'whoop' sound

   difficulty in breathing while coughing

   vomiting, particularly after a coughing bout

   disturbed sleep; tiredness; irritability; crying

Method

Baths

Dilute the following essential oils in 1 teaspoon vegetable oil:

thyme linalol – 3 drops
lavender – 1 drop
niaouli – 1 drop.

Add the diluted oil to the bath water, and swish around well before your child gets in.

Chest rub

Use a small amount of the following mix, over the chest and back, before sleep every night:

30 ml (1 ounce) almond oil
thyme linalol – 15 drops
ravensara – 15 drops
lavender – 20 drops.

Whooping cough mix
The following mix can be used in the two methods below. Follow the instructions in the boxes. First, mix the following:

thyme linalol – 10 drops
ravensara – 10 drops
eucalyptus radiata – 10 drops.

Steaming bowls
Put 10 drops of the whooping cough mix in a small bowl of steaming-hot water. Place the bowl in your child's room, somewhere out of reach of children and pets. Keep the door closed.

Pillow
At night, put 2 drops of the whooping cough mix on your child's pillow – on the underside, away from the eyes. It may stain, so use an old pillowcase.

To help with the coughing, prop your child upright on lots of extra pillows.

Essential oils that help

thyme linalol
eucalyptus radiata
ravensara
cypress
lavender
Dermatect (see 'Suppliers')

Professional aromatherapists may want to add one of the following three to this list: hyssopus decumbrens – add 2–3 drops to the whooping cough mix above; or (alternatively) add 4 drops of thymus vulgaris or 4 drops of origanum vulgare.

Other care

Fresh air is needed, so open a window. Use a humidifier in your child's room. Keep him or her away from atmospheric pollution, including cigarette smoke. Give your child lots to drink to rehydrate the body (see – Dehydration). Only give your child small meals, in case food is brought up during a bout of coughing. Fish, chicken and green vegetables are what's needed now – liquidized into a soup if that's the only way it'll get eaten. Also give your child vitamin C and cod-liver oil.

Mucus and phlegm will be coughed up. Keep a bowl nearby so your child can spit into it. Sterilize the bowl continually with boiling water and bleach.

Don't send your child back to school or nursery until you have your doctor's go-ahead.

When to get help

Whooping cough can be very serious in young children. Speak to your doctor immediately if you suspect whooping cough, especially if you know someone in the neighbourhood or school who has had it.

PREVENTION

   Inoculation is available; ask your doctor about vaccinations.

NINE

Aromatherapy for the Seriously Ill Child

There will always be children who have been loved and cared for, and even prayed for most intently, who will still become seriously ill and, tragically, some may not recover. Their parents will go through heart-breaking agony, often accompanied by feelings of guilt ('I didn't do enough'), fear ('What more pain will my child have to suffer?'), depression and sadness ('I cannot go on without my child'), and at the same time they're expected to be stoic and positive, for the sake of the child. Parents have told me they loathed the feeling of exclusion as they stood in corridors while strangers, the medical professionals, carried on their business around their child's bed.

We are very grateful to the doctors and nurses who care for our sick children, and there is no substitute for what they do. Many doctors these days are aiming to integrate conventional medical treatment with the best of the complementary therapies – what's called 'integrative medicine'. Aromatherapy is very much at the forefront of this trend, and not only because people find it so very pleasant, with its delicious aromas. Hospitals and hospices in many countries have trained aromatherapy staff on the premises. To suggest using a few essential oils on your child is not going to surprise many medical staff, as they've probably seen it done before.

Using essential oils on a sick child is one way to contribute toward their care. It does generally make children feel more comfortable: the lovely aromas lift the spirits and bring the richness of nature into the environment. As they allay fears and anxiety, they may introduce a new positivity.

It's fairly easy to use aromatherapy within a medical-care environment: essential oil sprays can be used in the atmosphere, and around bed linen: and, if the child is at home rather than a medical facility, a diffuser could be used.

When it comes to massage, you need medical clearance from your child's doctor. They will want to consider whether the delivery of drugs they've prescribed will be affected by the increased blood-flow. Each patient is different. It may be possible to massage your child's hands, or feet, arms, legs, or even their back. It may be more suitable to stroke their forehead or their head. A simple hand massage would be a good place to start, because it leads on so naturally from that thing all parents with sick children do – which is to sit by their child's bed and hold his or her hand. Just put a little oil on your child's hand and stroke it in gently, or massage very lightly.

Essential oils for the seriously ill child

rose otto	mandarin	The dilution rates are
neroli	tangerine	a third lower for sick
lemon	orange	children than for healthy
chamomile roman	geranium	children, unless carried
lavender	petitgrain	out by a professional.

Massage

Massage can increase blood-flow, and this can have an impact on the way carefully measured doses of drugs are delivered through the body – in chemotherapy, for example. For this reason, most institutions would prefer you to ask before attempting to massage your child.

By 'massage' I'm talking about very gentle upward movements, more like repeated stroking, on different parts of the body. If you are unsure, the hands and feet are a good place to start.

Room sprays

Essential oils can be used in room sprays to freshen up the stale air that is often present in hospitals, but don't let the water droplets fall on any electrical equipment. Choose from the suitable oils above – a little lavender can help a child to sleep. See Chapter 3 (page 15) for the quantities to use with different age groups and for method instructions.

Drug-dependent babies

I'll never forget hearing from a pediatric nurse that the worst thing for nurses caring for drug-dependent babies is witnessing the constant crying and screaming of innocent little souls going through withdrawal. Each baby is born with their particular set of symptoms and problems, possibly including infection with HIV. The nurses often feel helpless, and I know that for some it's just too much to cope with emotionally – especially as (for crack-dependent babies) the outlook is not always good. Of course, medication is given to these unfortunate children, as well as the best care – including being picked up, cuddled and soothed.

Aromatherapy can help in terms of emotional soothing and taking some of the edge off the harsh physical effects of withdrawal. A baby who has been subjected to narcotic drugs while in the womb, and who is now on medication, must be treated with a different set of rules to babies who haven't had to endure this unnatural assault on their system.

Drug-dependent babies

The following essential oils are suitable for use on drug-dependent babies.	lavender neroli chamomile roman rose otto	Each baby will have a smell preference which, with a little patience, you may discover.

With newborns, for whom the symptoms of withdrawal are worst, use 3 drops of essential oil, diluted in 15 ml (¹/2 ounce) almond oil. Gradually *reduce* the amount of essential oil over the following weeks, until the minimum amount of essential oil recommended for that age group is being used. Apply the diluted oil in a very gentle massage of the back, arms and legs. As these babies are always underweight, only a tiny amount will actually be used. Remember to be extremely gentle when applying the oil.

The same essential oil as used in the soothing massage can also be placed near the baby – just 1 drop placed on a tissue. The aroma will remind the baby of the love and care given to them with the gentle soothing massage, and will bring some reassurance and calm. Only use the same oil or blend of oils you are using in the massage, if it's been established through observation that the child is benefiting from it (signs to look for are less crying and greater calm).

Healing touch

In some forms of energy healing, the hands touch the body, whereas in others they do not. Strange as it may seem, just hovering the hands, palm down, about 2 inches from the surface of the body, can have a very calming effect, and can improve healing time. This 'no-hands' approach to healing can be useful when a child is on a drip, attached to other equipment, and generally in a delicate position. Simply place your hands in the air above your child, almost stroking the air around them, but not touching the body itself. If your child has a tummy pain, hold your hands above the tummy. If it's in the foot, put your hands there.

What follows is a brief outline of a particular healing method taught to nurses all over the world by Dolores Kreiger Ph.D, RN. It can be used by all parents, even those whose children are too sick to have physical contact.

First, get yourself comfortable and take a deep breath. Imagine your child at their funniest and most playful, when they were well. Keeping this image in your mind, imagine a band of energy, like the flow of a gentle stream, circling up the front of your child's body, and over the back in a neverending, continuous movement. Then see this flow as sparkling and full of light – rather like rippling water in bright sunlight. Now join the two images together – your happy, well child, and this sparkling flow of energy, or water, whichever is the easiest for you to imagine. See the sparkling stream flowing around your child in bed. This can be difficult at first, but take your time.

The next step is to put a hand into that imaginary flow of sparkling energy and gently hold it over the part of the body that seems to be the most problematic for your child at that particular time. Don't attempt to treat the illness itself – that is not your role here.

Now imagine your hand is getting full of soothing light. People will have different ideas about where the healing light comes from. Hold your hand there just for a few seconds at first, building up later to a longer period. As soon as your mind wanders, slowly take your hand away, leaving the sparkling energy in its place.

TEN

Mind, Mood and Emotion

Children suffer with negative states of mind, just as adults do. They too can feel stress, tension, anxiety, depression, guilt, shame and embarrassment. They too can lack self-confidence or self-esteem, and feel unworthy. Insecurity and fear may be in their mind. The pressures on children are different to the pressures on adults, but they are equally tough. We have work and bills to worry about, whereas they have homework every night and exams every year. While we have control over our lives, and can make decisions to change what is getting us down, children do not. And control, or the lack of it, is known from research to be one of the most important factors in the build-up of stress. Teenagers in particular have powerful peer pressure bending them this way and that, and the 'fashion police' to watch out for.

Sometimes, tragically, the pressures on children leads them to commit suicide as a means of escape. For others, escape may be found in drugs, drink or belonging to a gang. The mental state of our children is just as important as their physical state of health, but you can't measure self-esteem on a thermometer. You can see a rash and you can feel a swollen gland, but what happens inside a child's head is hidden.

There are many subjects that come under the general title 'mind, mood and emotion', and I have written about them at length in *The Fragrant Pharmacy* (what follows are a few brief suggestions from this book, which I have adapted here).

Alertness

Children have a great deal of studying to do, and it's a strain. Keeping the mind alert through lessons and homework is hard, especially when it's a subject the child has no interest in whatsoever. When a person studies, their mind is absorbing information. Often, the problem with exams is in actually being able to remember the information that was revised the night before – which is where essential oils come in. When your child is revising, they can use a particular essential oil nearby – in a diffuser, or on a tissue they can occasionally sniff – so the information studied then becomes associated with that particular aroma. When the exam comes along, your child can use that same aroma nearby – not in a diffuser, but on a tissue. They can discreetly sniff the aroma, which takes their mind back to study time and may help them recall the information. There are several rules to follow in this process:

    Try to use a fragrance the child has not used before, because an aroma used previously probably has associations that have nothing to do with the subject being absorbed. Or you could make a unique mix especially for each subject.

    If possible, use one fragrance (or mix) per subject, and not too much of it.

    Your child should only inhale the aroma when he or she needs to remember the studied information – in a test or exam, for example, and not at other times. If they use it all the time, their memory will get confused.

    Don't rely solely on this method. The aroma–memory connection is meant to be an additional aid, not a replacement for hard work. Your child can't just look at his or her textbooks expecting everything to go in magically. Sorry, it's not that easy: they'll have to put the time in and read their material thoroughly.

Children's alertness oils	Children's alertness mix
peppermint pine bergamot eucalyptus radiata lemon rosemary grapefruit lime	First, mix the following essential oils together. From this mix, take the appropriate number of drops for your child's age (see page 11). Use in the diffuser and tissue methods. grapefruit – 5 drops lime – 5 drops black pepper – 2 drops peppermint – 2 drops

Anxiety

You can guess your child is anxious if you find them sighing a lot, gasping for breath or needing to take in large chunks of air. It might even be that he or she is running to the toilet all the time, getting headaches or back pain, biting nails or just can't relax. Yet tiredness is common, as is restlessness, or even tremors. Anxiety can make people dizzy, perspire or blush, and it can raise blood pressure. A child might feel dry in the mouth, or belch a lot, feel nauseous, get diarrhoea or vomit. The stomach muscles can tighten up in a spasm, causing terrible pain. Anxiety causes stabbing pains in the chest, and stronger, faster heartbeats. It can make a child feel so unwell that his or her parents seriously wonder if there isn't something physical wrong.

Children's anxiety oils

bergamot
mandarin
neroli
rose otto
chamomile roman
geranium
frankincense

Children's anxiety mix

First, mix the following essential oils together. From this mix, take the appropriate number of drops for your child's age (see page 9). Use in baths, body oils, and all room methods.

bergamot – 5 drops
lavender – 1 drop
geranium – 3 drops

Stress

Children's stress can arise from exam pressure, emotional problems, peer pressure, home-life difficulties, school competition pressure, high parental expectations, feelings of being unable to cope, of helplessness and of everything being out of their control.

Symptoms include irritability, loss of sense of humour, difficulty in making decisions or concentrating or doing jobs in logical order, feeling defensive, angry inside and disinterested in large areas of life. Also, there may be insomnia, sweating, breathlessness, faints, loss of appetite and bingeing, indigestion, constipation or diarrhoea, headaches, cramps, muscle spasms, eczema, asthma, psoriasis and breathing problems.

Children's stress oils

lavender
ormenis flower
petitgrain
chamomile roman
geranium
mandarin
rose otto
neroli
ylang ylang

Children's stress mix

First, mix the following essential oils together. From this mix, take the appropriate number of drops for your child's age (see page 9). Use in baths, body oils, and all room methods.

chamomile roman – 5 drops
mandarin – 2 drops
ormenis flower – 3 drops
geranium – 3 drops

Suppliers

If you experience difficulty finding pure essential oils suitable for the purposes outlined in this book, the following aromatherapy dispensary/clinic can be recommended. The company has an international mail order service for essential oils, and natural products for children, babies and mothers-to-be:

Earth Garden
(essential oil and herbal dispensary)
2 Fairview Parade
Mawney Road
Romford
RM7 7HH

tel/fax 01708 722 633
or visit the Web site at *www.earthgarden.co.uk*

Please enclose a large stamped-addressed envelope for a product list.

Those who wish information to be sent outside of the UK, please enclose an international reply coupon (available at post offices).

Although it may not be possible to reply, the author is always pleased to read your personal healing stories. For details of workshops and seminars, write to the following address. Please enclose a stamped self-addressed envelope.

Valerie Ann Worwood
PO Box 38
Romford
RM1 1DN

Index